EEG Pearls

EEG Pearls

MARK QUIGG, MD, MSc

Director
Clinical EEG, Evoked Potential, and Intensive Monitoring Laboratories
F.E. Dreifuss Comprehensive Epilepsy Program
Associate Professor of Neurology
University of Virginia
Charlottesville, Virginia

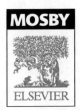

MOSBY

ELSEVIER

1600 John F. Kennedy Boulevard
Suite 1800
Philadelphia, PA 19103-2899

EEG PEARLS
ISBN-13: 978-0-323-04233-8

Copyright © 2006 by Mosby, Inc., an affiliate of Elsevier, Inc.
ISBN-10: 0-323-04233-3

Library of Congress Cataloging-in-Publication Data

EEG pearls / [edited by] Mark Quigg.–1st ed.
   p. ; cm.
  ISBN-13: 978-0-323-04233-8   ISBN-10: 0-323-04233-3
   1. Electroencephalography–Case studies.   2. Electroencephalography–Problems, exercises, etc.   I. Quigg, Mark.
   [DNLM: 1. Electroencephalography–Case Reports.
   2. Electroencephalography–Problems and Exercises.   3. Nervous System Diseases–diagnosis–Case Reports.   4. Nervous System Diseases–diagnosis–Problems and Exercises. WL 18.2 Q6e 2006]
   RC386.6.E43E13 2006
   616.8'047547–dc22

                                                      2006041975

ISBN-13: 978-0-323-04233-8
ISBN-10: 0-323-04233-3

Acquisitions Editor: Linda Belfus
Developmental Editor: Stan Ward
Project Manager: David Saltzberg

Printed and bound in the United Kingdom

Transferred to Digital Printing, 2011

CONTENTS

6. Fundamentals: Neonatal Polygraphy

7. Focal Sharp Transients and Localization-Related Epilepsy

8. Generalized Discharges and Generalized Epilepsy

9. Other Seizure Syndromes

Contents   **vii**

14. Status Epilepticus

For Lotta, Anders, and Erik

Acknowledgments

The author gratefully acknowledges the expert editorial assistance provided by the following colleagues:

HOWARD GOODKIN M.D., PH.D.
Assistant Professor of Neurology
University of Virginia
Charlottesville, Virginia

MARK A. GRANNER M.D.
Associate Professor of Clinical Neurology
Roy A. and Lucille J. Carver College of Medicine
University of Iowa
Iowa City, Iowa

WILLIAM R. HOBBS M.D.
Professor of Psychiatry
University of Virginia
Charlottesville, Virginia

JAMES Q. MILLER M.D.
Professor of Neurology
University of Virginia
Charlottesville, Virginia

The author also thanks the dedicated EEG technologists at the laboratory of the University of Virginia. Their high-quality work and helpful comments made this work possible.

Basic Electricity

Engineering advances allowed Hans Berger to record the first human electroencephalogram (EEG) in the late 1920s. Since then, EEG has evolved to become an important tool in the evaluation of epilepsy and encephalopathy.

The basic task of the EEG machine is the faithful detection of the electrical activities generated by the brain. Many details of the human EEG can be memorized. However, to understand EEG, to rationalize its behaviors, and to understand its confounders, an elementary knowledge of electricity and EEG technology is needed (Fig. 1-1).

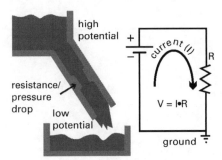

Figure 1-1. Basic science of electricity.

A *charge* (Q, coulomb) is the basic unit of electricity. One coulomb is equal to the total charge of $6 \bullet 10^{18}$ electrons.

Movement of electrons from place to place creates *current* (I, amperes, or amps). One amp (A) of current represents the flow of one coulomb of electrons during 1 s.

The electrical impetus that forces current from place to place is *voltage* or *potential* (V, volts). Voltage measures the energy applied to a unit of charge (V = energy/charge).

An analogy to water flow is a useful way to conceptualize electrical properties. Current flows "downhill" from regions of high gravitational potential to regions of low potential. Electrical potential is always measured as a comparison between two points. The electrical reference equivalent to atmospheric pressure at sea level is the *electrical ground*, the theoretical lowest potential within the substance of the earth.

The flow of current through a wire is impeded by *resistance* (Ω, ohms). The amount of current that can squeeze through a restriction—an electrical resistor—is related to the voltage that can be mustered to force it past the restriction. A small voltage can push a small current, and a large voltage can move a torrent. Similarly, a large resistor will cause a large drop in potential as current forces its way through, whereas a small resistor causes only a small loss. These relationships are represented by *Ohm's law*:

$$V = I \bullet R$$

Questions: 1. What is the term for the theoretical point of lowest potential?

2. What is the drop in potential at a 5 kΩ resistor for a current of 10 pA? Express the answer in units of μV.

3. What is the product of voltage and charge?

Answers: 1. The theoretical lowest potential is electrical ground. The measurement of electrical potential is always a comparison of potentials between two points.

2. $V = I \bullet R$

$$= 5 \text{ k}\Omega \bullet 10 \text{ pA}$$
$$= 5 \bullet 10^3 \Omega \bullet 10 \bullet 10^{-9} \text{ A}$$
$$= 50 \bullet 10^{-6} \text{ V}$$
$$= 50 \text{ μV}$$

3. Energy = voltage • charge

Pearls

1. Voltage is always measured as the difference in potential between two points.
2. $V = I \bullet R$ Voltage = current • resistance
3. Energy = voltage • charge

Elementary Circuits

When voltage remains constant for long periods of time, the current likewise remains constant. A common flashlight is an example of a direct current (DC) circuit, with a steady voltage supply (the battery) driving a constant current across the steady resistance of the flashlight bulb (Fig. 1-2).

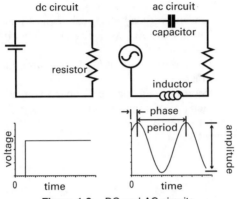

Figure 1-2. DC and AC circuits.

When voltage fluctuates over time, an alternating current (AC) circuit results. Household current in the United States alternates at a *frequency* of 60 cycles per second (cycles per second = Herz, or Hz). The *period* (analogous to wavelength) is the time from peak to peak of each cycle and is the reciprocal of frequency:

$$\text{Period} = 1/f$$

The *phase* is the reference point, usually the peak of the cycle, measured in relation to an initial point in time.

Household current oscillates rapidly between high and low potentials, in effect, pulling and pushing electrons back and forth. Most biologic signals form AC circuits, with the fluctuations of cations and anions moving across cell membranes playing the role of electrons oscillating within a wire.

The fluctuating nature of an AC circuit requires the addition of two circuit properties: *capacitance* and *inductance*. *Impedance* (Z, ohms, Ω) is the combined effect of capacitance, inductance, and resistance on AC current flow.

A *capacitor* consists of two conducting surfaces separated by a nonconducting insulator, such as a sandwich of two plates of metal separated by a rubber sheet. Inserted into a simple DC circuit, the capacitor allows the buildup of electrons on the plate nearest the voltage source until the mutual repulsion of the collected electrons begins to counterbalance the strength of the voltage source. Therefore, the flow of current gradually stops when the capacitor is "full." The more charge a capacitor can hold for a given voltage, the greater the *capacitance* (C, farad), given by the following equation:

$$C = Q/V$$
$$= \text{charge}/\text{voltage}$$

The effect of the capacitor is strikingly different when inserted into an AC circuit. As in the DC circuit, current flows until the capacitor is fully charged. However, when the AC power source fluctuates, and the potential pushing the electrons to the capacitor abruptly drops, the stored electrons are free to exit the capacitor in the opposite direction from which they entered. The current reverses direction. For an AC circuit, therefore, as long as the source of voltage fluctuates, a capacitor never totally blocks current flow, as it does in a DC circuit, because electrons continue to collect and disperse alternately on each side of the capacitor.

The contribution of capacitance to the overall impedance of an AC circuit depends on the frequency of the alternating current. The effective resistance of a capacitor to current flow is *capacitive reactance* (Xc) and is inversely proportional to the frequency and the capacitance:

$$Xc = 1/(2\pi \bullet f \bullet C)$$

Capacitive reactance to a current with a frequency of zero (a DC current) is infinite. As frequency increases, the capacitive reactance drops, allowing more current at the higher frequency to be pushed and pulled across the capacitor.

Inductance, although important in everyday electrical devices (electric motors are powered by induction of magnetism by fluctuating current), has negligible effect on EEG.

Questions: 1. What is the period of a current of 10 mA carried at a frequency of 50 Hz?
2. What constitutes a capacitor?
3. What is the relationship between frequency and capacitive reactance?
4. What is the capacitive reactance of a current with frequency of zero?
5. What is the impedance for a 25-Hz signal that generates 100 µV at a current of 0.02 mA? Express the answer in units of k.

Answers: 1. Period $= 1/f$
$= 1/50$ Hz
$= 0.02$ s
$= 20$ ms

2. A capacitor consists of two conducting surfaces separated by an insulator. In effect, any electrical junction between dissimilar materials can act as a capacitor. Capacitive reactance is important in EEG; one example is the impedance caused by the junction between the EEG electrode and the scalp. Oil, dirt, or dandruff, for example, could act as an insulator between the two conducting surfaces. Differences in impedance among electrodes can affect the quality of the recording.

3. $Xc = 1/f$. Note that signal frequency is also inversely proportional to the capacitance, a relationship essential in the design of EEG filters.

4. Capacitive reactance of a current with frequency of zero is infinite.

5. $Z = V/I$
$= 100$ µV/0.02 µA
$= 5000$ Ω
$= 5$ kΩ

Pearls

---

1. Resistance to current flow in an AC circuit is called *impedance* and is proportional to resistance and capacitive reactance.

2. Capacitive reactance is inversely proportional to frequency.

3. A capacitor is formed at any electrical junction. In the case of EEG, the most important contribution to impedance is the connection between scalp and electrode.

Electrical Safety

Any time two electrodes are attached to a subject and both electrodes are connected to a measuring device, the subject becomes a possible pathway for current. The safety of this biologic circuit element should not be taken for granted. Memorization of simple rules will keep everyone out of trouble.

First, electrical medical instruments must adhere to electrical safety requirements and must be inspected and approved by clinical engineering departments before use.

Second, medical instruments are grounded to earth. A defect in wiring, such as a frayed wire touching the metal instrument cabinet, can allow current to leak. Because current follows the path of least resistance, a good ground allows the current to flow away from, rather than through, the subject, who in contrast, offers a much higher resistance to current flow.

Third, the subject should not be exposed to *earth ground*. All electrical instruments that attach to the patient require a ground, from electrocardiogram (EKG) monitors to EEG machines to electrocautery devices. These instrument-patient connections are *isolated grounds;* in other words, although the subject and instrument achieve the same overall ground potential, the subject is not tied, in turn, to the main earth ground. Tying the subject to earth ground can be dangerous; the patient, in this case, becomes part of a low impedance circuit that can carry inadvertent current through the patient. Indeed, modern EEG systems totally isolate the patient from external current sources through a low capacitance barrier, through optical-electrical transducers, or other engineering means.

Fourth, the subject should not be exposed to multiple grounds. Although ground denotes the lowest possible electrical potential, the ground potential at one location may not exactly coincide with another at all times. When our sea level analogy to ground potential is applied, small waves come and go that minutely change the level of water. The presence of two grounds, either through differences in impedance in their connection to the body or by fluctuations in ground potentials among different sources, can allow current to flow from ground to ground. Different instruments, therefore, connect to a common patient ground. Another advantage of a common ground is that, often, electrical noise is minimized, enabling a clean recording.

Question: What is the artifact of the tracing below (Fig. 1-3) at electrode F3? Note that because channels Fp1-F3 and F3-C3 share a common faulty electrode, the noise it generates will appear in both.

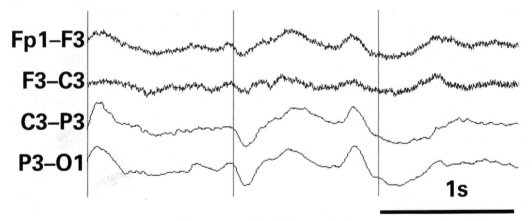

Figure 1-3. Artifact at electrode F3.

Answer: 60 Hz electrical artifact.

Pearls

1. All medical devices must be approved by an appropriate clinical engineering department.

2. Avoid multiple grounds, both to avoid noise marring the recording and to minimize the possibility of electrocution.

Filters

EEG machines use filters to dampen extraneous potentials. Before computerization and the advent of the digital EEG, filters were constructed from combinations of capacitors and resistors (Fig. 1-4).

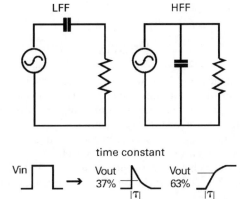

Figure 1-4. Low-frequency and high-frequency filters.

The key to understanding filters is to recall the relationship between signal frequency and capacitive reactance. It takes time for a capacitor to store up or discharge current, a duration measured by the *time constant* (τ in seconds). For any given resistance R and capacitance C, $\tau = R \cdot C$.

Capacitors charge or discharge at an exponential rate. Whereas biologists use half-life to describe exponential relationships, engineers use the natural logarithm e. The time constant for an RC circuit is the duration required for the output signal to discharge to 37% ($1/e$) of the input signal. In succinct mathematical terms, for an RC circuit in which Vo = output voltage and Vi = input voltage:

$$Vo = Vi \cdot e^{-t/\tau}$$

A *low-frequency filter* (LFF, sometimes called a high-pass filter) uses a capacitor wired in series with a resistor. High-frequency signals can pass through the capacitor because the capacitive reactance is small for rapidly alternating currents. Low frequencies, on the other hand, are more easily blocked because capacitive reactance rises with decreasing frequency. Low-frequency filters remove low frequency artifact, such as potentials generated from slight temperature changes or skin conductance (galvanic potentials), tissue-electrode polarization, and patient movement.

A *high-frequency filter* (HFF, or low-pass filter) uses a capacitor wired in parallel with a resistor. High-frequency signals preferentially shunt through the capacitor because the capacitive reactance is small in comparison to resistance. Conversely, low-frequency signals "see" a large capacitive reactance and proceed along the easier path through the resistor. High-frequency filters remove artifact, such as muscle noise from the signal.

A *notch filter* uses combinations of RC circuits to remove specific frequencies from a signal. The typical application for a notch filter is the removal of 60-Hz electrical noise from the signal.

The signals for display in digital EEG also undergo filtering, but RC circuits are replaced by mathematical functions that manipulate frequency spectra. Nevertheless, most manufacturers maintain terminology and function derived from traditional analog recording methods.

Questions: 1. What is the relationship between resistance, capacitance, and time constant in an RC circuit?
2. The time constant measures the time it takes for a capacitor to discharge by what percentage of its initial value?

3. Does an HFF remove high frequencies by putting a capacitor in series or in parallel with a resistor?

Answers: 1. $\tau = R \bullet C$

2. 37% of discharge. Note that τ also designates the time a capacitor charges to 63% of the maximum voltage.

3. Parallel.

Pearls

1. The time constant measures how long an RC circuit takes to charge and discharge a capacitor, with longer time constants implying larger capacitors that offer a lower capacitive reactance. Thus, the shorter the time constant, the more difficulty low-frequency signals will have traversing an RC circuit.

2. Low-frequency filters have a capacitor in series with a resistor and remove low-frequency signals. The standard setting for LFF is 1 Hz.

3. High-frequency filters have a capacitor in parallel with a resistor and remove high-frequency signals. The standard settings for HFF are 70 Hz or 35 Hz (varies with manufacturer).

Filters and Cutoff Frequency

The amount of filtering applied to an EEG signal is specified by the filter's *cutoff frequency* (f_{cutoff}) or time constant (τ). Traditionally, time constant and cutoff frequency are interchangeably used to designate the LFF setting, whereas the cutoff frequency designates the HFF setting. The cutoff frequency can be calculated from the time constant by the following equation:

$$f_{cutoff} = (\pi/2) \bullet 1/\tau$$

In the tracing in Figure 1-5, different filter settings are applied to the same signal. Manufacturers designate the cutoff frequency settings on their EEG machines by noting the setting at which 70% of the signal at the cutoff frequency passes through the filter. For example, an LFF setting of 1 Hz denotes that frequencies = 1 Hz will be attenuated by at least 30%, and frequencies <1 Hz will be attenuated even further at an exponential rate. An HFF of 70 Hz denotes that frequencies = 70 Hz will be attenuated by 30% or more. Sometimes the cutoff level of 70% is represented in decibels (db):

$$db = 20 \bullet \log(Vout/Vin)$$

A cutoff limit of 70% translates to -3 db.

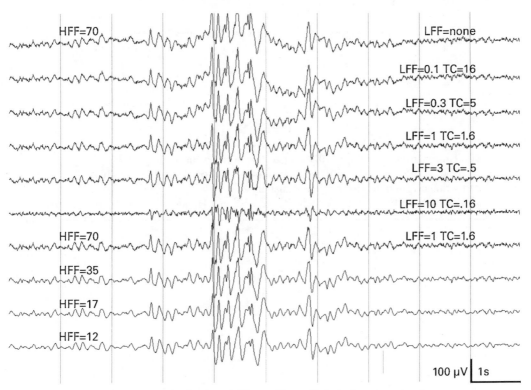

Figure 1-5. Application of different filter settings to the same signal.

The tracing in Figure 1-5 shows a burst of fast spike-wave discharges. Note that, with the LFF set to OFF, the signal "clips" and goes beyond the bounds allowed for the channel because the baseline is susceptible to low-frequency deviations. With the LFF set to 10 Hz, however, nearly all activity other than sharp waves are attenuated. An LFF setting of 1 Hz is the standard setting. The standard LFF setting of 1 Hz (t = 0.16 s) increases readability by removing the tendency for the tracing to wander from a flat baseline, while preserving low-frequency detail.

Filters and Cutoff Frequency

With the HFF set to 70 Hz, there is a slight "fuzziness" of the signal due to minimal electrical noise. Conversely, an HFF setting of 12 Hz severely comprises the morphology of the signal, blunting the sharpness of the epileptiform discharges. Standard settings for HFF are 70 Hz or 35 Hz.

Questions: 1. What are the standard LFF and HFF settings for routine EEG?
2. Which *f*cutoff filter setting removes the lowest frequency signal: LFF = 10 Hz, LFF = 0.1 Hz, or LFF = 1 Hz?

Answers: 1. LFF = 1 Hz, HFF = 70 Hz or 35 Hz.
2. LFF = 10 Hz. At this setting, frequencies at 10 Hz or slower are attenuated >30%.

Such relationships are easily summarized by a frequency-response graph (Fig. 1-6) that plots the rate of attenuation of output signal at different filter settings.

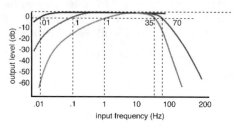

Figure 1–6. Frequency-response curve.

Pearls

1. Time constant is reciprocally related to the filter cutoff frequency.
2. The cutoff frequency indicates the frequency above or below which 70% of the input voltage is allowed to pass on to display.
3. Routine starting cutoff frequencies are LFF = 1 Hz and HFF = 70 Hz or 35 Hz.

Basic Principles of Electricity

Sensitivity and Paper Speed

Sensitivity defines the amplitude of the EEG display signal: how large a given EEG potential displays upon the paper or computer screen (Fig. 1-7). Analog and digital EEG systems differ in the units of sensitivity.

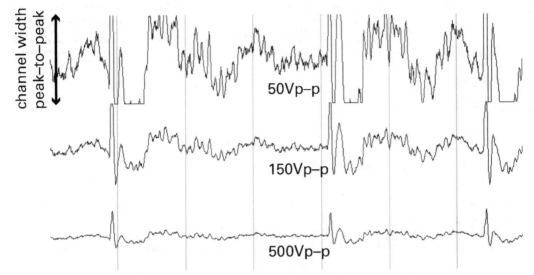

Figure 1-7. Sensitivity defines the amplitude of the EEG display signal.

The units of sensitivity of an analog EEG system are given in $\mu V/mm$, thus enabling the interpreter to easily calculate the amplitude of a potential by measuring its height in millimeters and multiplying by the sensitivity value. For example,

$$\text{Potential} \, (\mu V) = \text{height} \, (mm) \bullet \text{sensitivity} \, (\mu V/mm)$$
$$= 10 \text{ mm} \bullet 7 \, \mu V/mm$$
$$= 70 \, \mu V$$

Digital EEG systems divide the display into the number of vertical pixels allowed for each channel. The units of sensitivity of a digital EEG system are given in peak-to-peak (p-p) microvolts per channel. A sensitivity of 150 μV p-p, therefore, specifies that the maximum potential fully visible in that channel is 150 μV.

The trade-off for the ease in measurement is that the number designating sensitivity is reciprocal to its effect; in other words, the same signal displayed at a sensitivity of 10 $\mu V/mm$ (or its approximate digital equivalent of 300 μV p-p) will be displayed smaller than it would be at a sensitivity of 2 $\mu V/mm$ (or around 50 μV p-p).

Sensitivity, analogous to the volume level of a stereo, has no inherently correct value and is set best to display potentials at the most informative level. Usually, the level appropriate for most adult studies is 7 $\mu V/mm$ (or 150 μV p-p). Sensitivities that are too high cause *blocking* (so-called because the sweep of the EEG pens allows them to hit one another) or *clipping* (in the case of digital EEG) and are to be avoided in recording of high-amplitude potentials. The EEG technologist must label the tracing whenever changing sensitivity so that the interpreter makes no mistakes in comparing the amplitudes of potentials across different sections. For scalp recordings, the maximum sensitivity is 2 $\mu V/mm$; signals with amplitude below 1 mm at this setting are considered noise.

Standard *paper speed* of EEG recordings in the United States is 30 mm/s (Fig. 1-8). Faster speeds of 60 mm/s are sometimes used intermittently during a tracing to closely examine high-frequency activity or closely spaced potentials. Slower paper speeds of 15 mm/s allow conservation of paper and

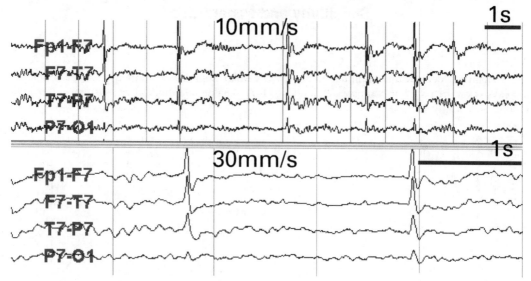

Figure 1-8. Paper speeds of 10 mm/s and 30 mm/s (standard speed in the United States).

facilitate the study of slower frequencies. Digital EEG systems allow changing of these parameters (as well as others) on the fly.

Most EEG systems, paper or digital, display EEG as 10-second pages, with major divisions denoting 1 s and 5 minor subdivisions of 200 ms each. Examples in this book omit minor divisions for clarity.

Questions: 1. What is the amplitude in µV of a signal measured on a paper EEG with height = 7 mm at a sensitivity of 7 µV/mm?
2. What is the maximum sensitivity of a standard tracing?

Answers: 1. Amplitude = measurement • sensitivity
= 7 mm • 7 µV/mm
= 49 µV

Most calibration signals for analog EEGs are 50 µV; therefore, the calibration signal measures around 7 mm at the standard sensitivity of 7 µV/mm.
2. The traditional maximum limit of sensitivity is 2 µV/mm. At this sensitivity on scalp recordings, signals below 1 mm in amplitude are considered noise.

Pearls

---

1. Sensitivity determines the display size of signals on paper (analog µV/mm) or on the display screen (µV p-p).
2. The standard sensitivity for analog tracings is 7 µV/mm, and the maximum is 2 µV/mm.
3. Standard paper speed is 30 mm/s displayed in 10-second pages.
4. Technologists must annotate the tracing so that changes in sensitivity, filter settings, paper speed, or montages are clearly observable by the interpreter.

REFERENCE
1. American Electroencephalographic Society. Guideline one: Minimum technical requirements for performing clinical electroencephalography. J Clin Neurophysiol 1994; 11:2–5.

Signal Processing

Digital EEG is rapidly becoming the standard in American clinical neurophysiology laboratories. The advantages in storage, data analysis, and display over traditional analog systems will become evident with the examples in this book. An understanding of analog-to-digital (ATD) conversion is necessary to understand limitations of this technique.

Analog data, the traditional voltage-time data displayed by the EEG, are smoothly and continuously variable. Digital data, on the other hand, are converted into discrete, stepped values. The finer the steps, the more accurately digital data represent analog data. Two variables, sampling frequency and bit depth, determine the accuracy of ATD conversion (Fig. 1-9).

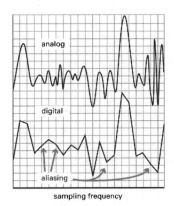

sampling frequency

Figure 1-9.   Analog and digital signal processing.

Sampling frequency determines the number and density of samples taken along the time axis. A sampling frequency of 100 Hz, therefore, reads 100 values for voltage data consecutively for each second of data. Sampling frequency determines the size of data files: a sampling frequency of 200 Hz is more accurate than 100 Hz but creates data files twice the size. The accuracy of sampling is limited by *Nyquist's theorem:*

$$\text{Sampling frequency} = 2 \bullet f_{\max}$$

In other words, the fastest frequency signal that can accurately be represented is one-half the sampling frequency. For example, a sampling frequency of 256 Hz accurately represents signal frequencies up to 128 Hz. *Aliasing* occurs when high-frequency signals are misrepresented as slower-frequency signals because they are undersampled.

Bit depth, sometimes referred to as *vertical resolution,* designates the number of divisions into which the range of voltages can be represented. Because computer memory is binary-based, each stepwise increase in bit depth increases the number of possible amplitude levels by a factor of 2. For example, a bit depth of 8 means that there are $2^8 = 256$ individual steps between the minimum and maximum allowable voltages. A bit depth of 9 provides an amplitude resolution of $2^9 = 512$.

Question: 1. Given that the clinically relevant range of EEG frequencies is about 0.5–30 Hz, what is the minimum appropriate sampling frequency for routine digital EEG?

Answer: 1. Trick question. By Nyquist's theorem, to accurately represent signals of 30 Hz, the minimum sampling frequency is 60 Hz. However, the range of clinically relevant EEG frequencies is a different question from the range necessary to represent the morphology of EEG signals accurately. A sampling frequency of 60 Hz limits the shortest duration that can be accurately measured to the reciprocal of $60 = 1/60 = 0.01667$ s ≈ 17 ms. Because some interictal epileptiform discharges have durations of approximately 20 ms, a sampling frequency of 60 Hz could completely miss some discharges or render others as jagged steps in the tracing.

Digital EEG systems use sampling frequencies between 100 and 500 Hz. A typical bit depth is usually 16 ($2^{16} = 65536$, or in the common computer convention, 64k).

Pearls

1. The highest accurately portrayed frequency in a digital EEG is one-half the sampling rate.
2. Increasing bit depth or vertical resolution of digital data by one step requires a doubling of storage media.

The Differential Amplifier

An *amplifier* is a device that receives an input signal, guides a power source, and creates an amplified copy of the original signal. The increase in voltage is called *gain* and is calculated from the ratio of the output and input voltages. Often gain is expressed as the engineering term *decibels* (db):

$$db = 20 \bullet \log{(Vout/Vin)}$$

Thus, a gain of one magnitude (Vout/Vin = 10) is 20 db, two magnitudes (Vout/Vin = 100) = 40 db.

Most amplifiers used in recordings of biologic signals are a combination of amplifiers called a *differential amplifier*. The output of a differential amplifier is the amplified difference between two inputs, called *G1* and *G2*. ("G" comes from the days when the electrical contacts to tube amplifiers were grids) (Fig. 1-10). The main benefit of the differential amplifier is noise reduction, quantified by the term *common mode rejection*. Any voltage seen in common between G1 and G2 adds up to zero and thereby cancels out. One can calculate the *common mode rejection ratio* (CMRR) by shorting G2 to ground and taking the ratio of the input and output signals. The higher the CMRR, typically 10^5, the better the quality of the differential amplifier.

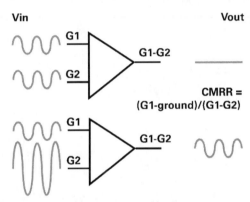

Figure 1-10. The output of a differential amplifier is the amplified difference between two inputs, called *G1* and *G2*.

Common mode rejection works most effectively if the impedances of inputs at G1 and G2 are equally matched. In the example, noise, represented as the sinusoidal input signal, is recorded with equal voltages at G1 and G2 because the impedances of G1 and G2 are similar. In this case, noise cancels out. In the case of *impedance mismatching*, the "bad electrode" at G2 records noise at a higher voltage than G1. Because G1 and G2 transmit unequal voltages, the noise no longer cancels out. The recommended maximum impedance of scalp electrodes in EEG is 5kΩ.

Questions: 1. What is the amplification factor for an amplifier with a gain of 120 db?
2. What is the maximum scalp electrode impedance in EEG?
3. What are the designators for inputs to a differential amplifier?

Answers: 1. Gain: db $= 20 \bullet$ log (Vout/Vin)

$\qquad\qquad$ 120 db $= 20 \bullet$ log (Vout/Vin)

$\qquad\qquad$ 6 $=$ log (Vout/Vin)

$\qquad\qquad$ $10^6 =$ Vout/Vin

2. Maximum scalp electrode impedance $= 5$ kΩ

3. G1 and G2 are the designators of the inputs to a differential amplifier.

Pearls

1. Gain is the amplification factor of differential amplifiers, often measured in db.

2. Common mode rejection is the noise-reduction design of the differential amplifier. The higher the common mode rejection ratio, the better.

3. G1 and G2 are the names given by convention for each input pair of electrodes of the differential amplifier.

4. Because impedance mismatch can cause amplification of degraded signal, the maximum impedance of scalp electrodes in EEG is 5kΩ.

Electroencephalographic Electrodes

The collection of data from the patient to the electroencephalographic (EEG) machine starts at the EEG electrode. Soo Ik Lee (MD, former director of the EEG laboratory at the University of Virginia) believed that bad electrodes are like bad teenagers. They either distort the truth or completely make up stories when it suits them. If left uncorrected, they get worse. Similarly, bad electrodes distort brain electrical activity and create their own signals if mismanaged, and only get worse if untended.

The goal of electrode placement and maintenance is to make the conduction of electrical current from scalp to machine as accurate as possible.

The process starts at the scalp with a scrubbing of the electrode site with a pumice-laced detergent that lightly abrades the skin and removes oil. A conductive gel containing salts in a viscous medium is applied so that ions can carry current between the electrode and skin. *Silver-chloride* electrodes, named so because the silver has been purposely oxidized with a chloride solution, facilitate conversion of ionic current flow to electron current flow. Silver and chloride ions on the electrode surface are free to pass into the gel solution. However, an oil layer left on the scalp that separates skin and gel creates the equivalent of a large capacitor (two conductors separated by an insulator). A capacitor in the current path raises impedance of the electrode, artificially increasing its signal relative to its neighbors (impedance mismatch). The capacitor also acts as a low-frequency filter, further distorting signal. Scalp electrodes should have a maximum impedance of <5 kΩ (Fig. 2-1).

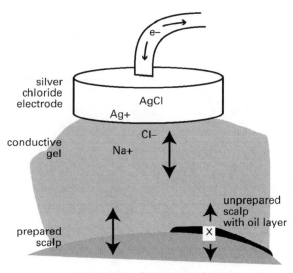

Figure 2-1. Scalp electrodes.

During intermittent photic stimulation (an activation procedure intended to induce abnormalities susceptible to flashing lights), high impedance can cause significant *photoelectric responses*. In this situation, the minute current generated by photons striking a salt-metallic battery (the electrode and conductive gel) is amplified by high impedances to generate visible potentials.

Impedances that are too low can also cause signal distortion. A *salt bridge* results when the patient's sweat, messy electrode gel, or wet hair allows current flow from electrode to electrode, thus "short-circuiting" the electrode pair. The low impedance between the pair allows the transmission of low-frequency artifact into the channel.

Electrodes are held in place with the use of tape, the viscosity of the gel, or special electrode systems that use "bathing caps." Longer-term electrodes are glued in place with collodion, a flammable compound related to gunpowder that requires ether or acetone for its removal. Some centers, faced with difficulties in ventilation, have experimented with cyanoacrylate glues (Superglue) for long-term electrode placement.

Bimetallic artifact results when excess electrode gel bridges the junction between the silver of the electrode and the copper of the wire; the dissimilar metals joined by a conductive gel create a small battery that can inject current into the signal path.

A good technologist will control these potential problems and comment during the tracing on any identification of artifact and its correction. Factors that might influence electrode problems (poor hygiene, scalp wounds, skull defects, and patient position laying upon certain electrodes) should also be documented to enable proper interpretation.

Question: How might scalp edema affect EEG signal?

Answer: Scalp edema may increase the distance between cortex and electrode, thus decreasing the intensity of the electrical signal. Fluid collections that increase cortex-electrode distance, such as subdural hematomas or hygromas, cause the most striking decrements in signal. Scalp edema has no predictable effects on impedance itself, unless scalp preparation was limited because of friability of skin.

Clinical Pearls

---

1. Scalp electrodes are commonly constructed of discs of silver prepared with chloride salts.

2. Electrode placement requires scalp cleaning, abrasion, and electrical contact with the use of a conductive gel.

3. Neatness counts: Patient hygiene, sweating, excess or sparse electrode gel, and poor scalp preparation all may adversely affect electrode impedance.

4. The EEG technologist must document identification of electrode artifacts and their attempted correction.

10–20 System

The placement of electrodes on the scalp is based on the *International 10–20 System*. Four cardinal points are determined from head anatomy: the nasion (the indentation of the nose between the eyes), the inion (the midline occipital protuberance), and the left and right preauricular points (indentations just anterior to the ear). These points determine the sagittal and coronal midlines. "10–20" refers to the percentages of lengths determined from the two midlines (Fig. 2-2). By basing electrode locations on percentages rather than fixed distances, the relationships between skull anatomy and underlying brain regions are maintained for a broad range of head sizes.

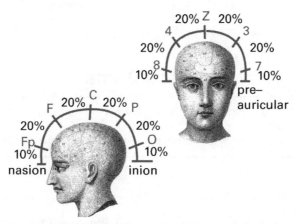

Figure 2-2. The International 10–20 System for placement of electrodes on the scalp.

Note that electrodes overlie specific anatomic regions: the left anterior temporal region (T1, F7, T7), the right posterior parietal region (P3), and the central vertex (Cz). Although these regions correspond to brain anatomy, the fact that scalp electrodes record from a volume of underlying brain means that one cannot name EEG regions as emanating from a specific brain focus (Fig. 2-3). For example, it is overambitious to say that a focal discharge was seen in the "left midtemporal lobe"; the correct designation is the "left midtemporal region."

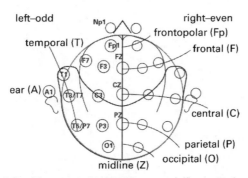

Figure 2-3. Placement of electrodes on specific anatomic regions.

Electrode sites are named according to the 10–20 grid. For example, "F3" refers to the frontal coronal plane and the left-sided 20% sagittal plane. Numbers increase from the midline out, odd numbers designating the left and even right. Naming conventions, until recently, have differed somewhat between the United States and other countries. U.S. labs tended to persist in the use of an older standard in which electrodes overlying the temporal region are prefixed "T" with the number increasing anteriorly to posteriorly. EEGs in this book adhere to the international naming convention.

Some electrodes fall outside the standard 10–20 grid. *True temporal* electrodes (T1 and T2) are placed 1 cm above and 1/3 the distance of the line joining the external auditory meatus to the external canthus. *Ear electrodes* (A1 and A2) are attached to the ear lobe. Nasopharyngeal electrodes are Z-shaped, blunt-tipped wires that are inserted into the nose and turned so that the ends contact the soft palate, a placement designed to record activity from the basal frontal and mesial structures.

Question: What is the distance, in percentage distance, separating F3 from O1?

Answer: 60%; 20% from F3 to C3, 20% from C3 to P3, 20% from P3 to O1.

Clinical Pearls

1. Scalp electrodes are placed and named according to the International 10–20 System.
2. Scalp electrodes record from brain regions, not from specific lobes.

REFERENCES

1. Jasper HH: Report of the Committee on Methods of Clinical Examination in Electroencephalography. Electroencephalogr Clin Neurophysiol 1957; 10:370.
2. Klem G, Luders H, Jasper H: The ten-twenty electrode system of the International Federation of Clinical Neurophysiology. Electroencephalogr Clin Neurophysiol 1999; 52:3–6.

Channels and Montages

Electrical potential is a relative measurement; therefore, voltage is always calculated as the difference in potential between two points. Accordingly, a *channel* in EEG is the display of the difference in potential from two inputs. By convention, these two inputs are labeled G1 and G2. A channel is defined, by convention, by listing the input to G1 first and to G2 second. For example, F8-T8 designates a channel with electrode F8 at G1 and T8 at G2.

The *pen rule* determines which way the display swings to define the difference in potential between G1 and G2 for each channel (Fig. 2-4). Long ago, electroencephalographers decided that if the potential at G1 is more positive than the potential at G2, then the pen (or in modern days, the line on the computer monitor) swings down. If G2 is more positive than G1, then the pen swings up. An easy way to remember the convention is that, in effect, the pen always swings to the more negative electrode.

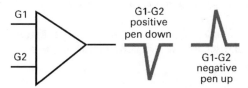

Figure 2-4. The pen rule determines which way the display swings to define the difference in potential between G1 and G2 for each channel.

Montages define the topographic display of EEG channels. The two main types of montages are *bipolar* and *referential* (Fig. 2-5).

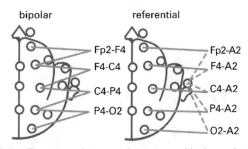

Figure 2-5. The two main types of montages: bipolar and referential.

The channels of *bipolar* montages are constructed from chains of pairs of adjacent electrodes. A *longitudinal bipolar montage* consists of chains that run in the sagittal orientation. A *transverse bipolar* montage consists of chains that run in the coronal orientation. Bipolar montages have two main strengths. First, focal discharges are relatively easy to pick out from ongoing background activity. Second, recording from active, awake individuals is facilitated because movement artifact, tending to be present equally among all electrodes, tends to cancel out, acting in concert with the common mode rejection present at each differential amplifier. The weakness of bipolar montages is that, because of the "common mode rejection" quality, they can also distort generalized cerebral activity.

The channels of *referential montages* consist of G1 inputs attached to scalp electrodes and G2 inputs attached to a common reference electrode. Referential montages work best when the reference electrode is indifferent, meaning that it is "blind" to or uninvolved in the ongoing activity of interest. The reference electrode can be an actual, single electrode, such as the ear pictured previously, or an electrical or mathematical construct. For example, to decrease artifact, reference inputs can be

Channels and Montages   **21**

constructed by joining both ears (A1 + A2), by averaging all cerebral inputs (all average), or by calculating a weighted average in favor of nearby electrodes (a Laplacian reference). The strength of referential montages is their ability to accurately render generalized or diffuse activity. The weakness of referential montages lies in that they are only as good as the chosen reference. Loss of the reference (such as in the active or uncooperative patient) means loss of the recording. Involvement of the reference by artifact or by focal activity colors all channels. Furthermore, use of a common reference results in various interelectrode distances. The farther one electrode is from another, the more relative amplification of signal between the electrodes results. For example, if electrodes T1 and T2 are referenced to the left ear, channel T1-A1 will show a smaller pen deflection than T2-A1 for the same input potential.

Montages are analogous to different cuts on neuroimaging, and, like neuroimaging, no study is complete without assessing different views. EEG standards require a minimum of three montages for standard EEG: one longitudinal bipolar, one transverse bipolar, and one referential. Digital EEG has the distinct advantage of the ability to reformat data into various montages ''on the fly,'' a property used in later examples.

A montage should be explicitly labeled on the tracing, either by sketching it prior to each montage switch or by labeling each channel with its inputs.

Questions: 1.   What montage is shown on the tracing in Figure 2-6?
2.   What polarity is the discharge shown between the arrows?

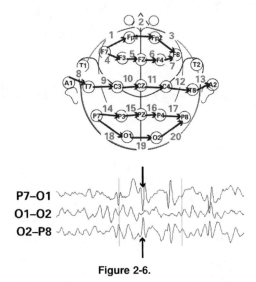

Figure 2-6.

Acquisition of the Electroencephalogram

Answers: 1. Montage = transverse bipolar.

2. The polarity of the sharp discharge at the arrow is negative. In this example, channel P7-O1 points downwards, therefore G2 must be more negative than G1. Channel O2-P8 points upward, thus G1 must be more negative than G2. Therefore, the polarity of the discharge between C3 and C4 must be negative. Phase-reversal of waveforms is the method of localization of focal discharges used for bipolar montages. Note that channel O1-O2 hardly deflects at all, indicating that G1 and G2 are equally involved in the field of the electrical potential.

Clinical Pearls

1. Every channel is made of two inputs, G1 and G2.
2. If G1 > G2 (G2 more negative), then there is a downward deflection in the channel.
3. If G1 < G2 (G1 more negative), then there is an upward deflection in the channel.
4. Three montages (longitudinal and transverse bipolars, referential) are required for every standard EEG.

REFERENCE

1. American Electroencephalographic Society: Guideline one: Minimum technical requirements for performing clinical electroencephalography. J Clin Neurophysiol Electroencephalographic Society 1994; 11:2–5.

Localization 1

Localization is the process of identifying the polarity and location of an EEG finding. Localization is possible with scalp EEG because of an important simplification. For all of the complex structures of gyri, sulci, and fissures of the brain, its electrical properties can be represented as a smooth hemisphere.

This model has several important implications. First, although all electrical potentials form dipoles with one end positive and the other negative, often scalp electrodes only record from one half of the dipole; the other half projects to the lower hemisphere and is not recordable. Second, because the brain has a complex structure, potentials that occur within certain regions may occur without showing on the scalp. For example, the base of the frontal lobe, because it is relatively far away from scalp electrodes, may harbor occult potentials.

In the examples below, the electrical dipole is represented as a + or −. Isopotential lines drawn on the scalp designate regions with equal polarity that drop in intensity with distance from the source. Such maps define an *electrical field*, the distribution of influence that an individual discharge imparts upon a conductive volume. The EEG for each potential is shown in two montages, a longitudinal bipolar and a referential to an ear.

In Figure 2-7, a negative potential occurs nearest T8. In the longitudinal montage, channels Fp2-F8 and F8-T8 show downward deflections because, in each case, G2 of each channel is more negative than G1. The amplitude of the deflection is greater in F8-T8 because the potential is nearer and stronger at that location, whereas channel Fp2-F8, being farther away, records a weaker potential. Conversely, channels T8-P8 and P8-O2, in amplitudes reflecting their distance from the discharge, show upward deflections because G1 of each pair is more negative than G2. This pattern of opposite deflections, channels pointing out-of-phase, is called *phase reversal*. Phase reversal is the main means of identifying the location of a focal discharge with bipolar montages.

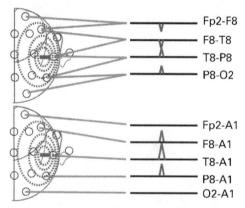

Figure 2-7. Phase reversal is the main means of identifying the location of a focal discharge with bipolar montages.

In the referential montage, the right scalp electrodes are referred to the left ear. All channels deflect upward because the negative potential at T8 renders G1 of each pair more negative than the common reference A1. The amplitude of deflection increases with the proximity of the electrode to the focal discharge. Amplitude is the main means of identifying the location of a focal discharge with referential montages.

Question: Predict the pattern of deflections in the EEG caused by the negative discharge at P8 in Figure 2-8.

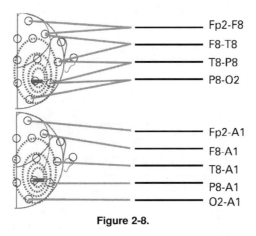

Figure 2-8.

Answer: In the bipolar montage, an upward deflection in channel P8-O2 indicates that G1 (P8) is more negative than G2 (O2). Channels T8-P8 and F8-T8 deflect downward because G1 is less negative than G2 (Fig. 2-9). Channel Fp2-F8 is isopotential (no deflection) because both inputs carry the same potential. In the referential montage, the highest upward deflection is at P8, indicating that G1 is strongly more negative than G2. Smaller upward deflections occur in nearby electrodes.

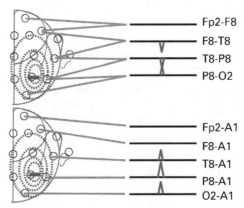

Figure 2-9. Channels T8-P8 and F8-T8 deflect downward because G1 is less negative than G2.

Clinical Pearls

1. Phase-reversal is the main means of identifying the location of a focal discharge with bipolar montages.
2. Amplitude is the main means of identifying the location of a focal discharge with referential montages.

Localization 2

Questions: Continue predicting the pattern of EEG deflections induced by the following discharges.

1. See Figure 2-10.

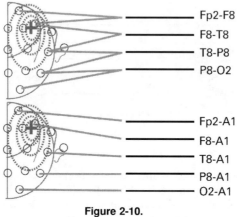

Figure 2-10.

2. See Figure 2-11.

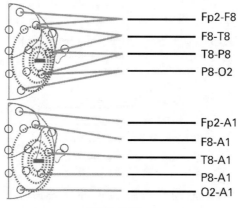

Figure 2-11.

Acquisition of the Electroencephalogram

3. See Figure 2-12.

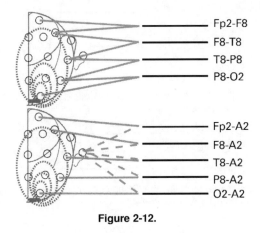

Figure 2-12.

Answers: 1. This example shows a positive potential nearest F8. Note that the direction of deflections for the positive discharge is opposite that of a negative discharge (Fig. 2-13).

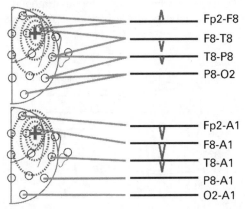

Figure 2-13. Note that the direction of deflections for the positive discharge above is opposite that of a negative discharge.

2. This example shows the result of a negative discharge equally spaced between electrodes T8 and P8; channel T8-P8 in the bipolar montage is isopotential. A phase reversal, however, is still present in channels F8-T8 and P8-O2. Therefore, a phase reversal in a bipolar montage need not occur in adjacent channels. The referential montage, reflecting that P8 and O2 are equally involved, shows that the amplitude of the negative discharge is equal in both T8-A2 and P8-A2 (Fig. 2-14).

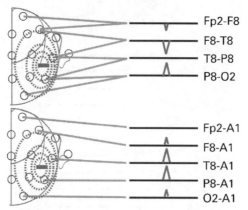

Figure 2-14. The referential montage, reflecting that P8 and O2 are equally involved, shows that the amplitude of the negative discharge is equal in both T8-A2 and P8-A2.

3. Figure 2-12 shows a negative discharge that occurs somewhat posterior to electrode O2, a location termed *end-of-chain*. In an end-of-chain discharge, the expected phase reversal in the bipolar montage does not occur because there is no electrode on the other side to straddle over the focal potential. Therefore, each G1-G2 pair records that G2 is more negative than G1. Each channel, as a result, deflects downward. On the other hand, in the referential montage G1 from each pair is more negative than G2, and each channel deflects upward in proportion to its distance from the occipital potential (Fig. 2-15).

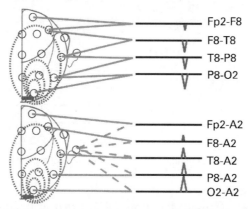

Figure 2-15. In the referential montage G1 from each pair is more negative than G2, and each channel deflects upward in proportion to its distance from the occipital potential.

Clinical Pearls

1. Isopotential channels can result from either being equally uninvolved by a focal discharge or from being equally involved.
2. Focal discharges that occur at the end-of-chain may show no phase reversal on a bipolar montage.

Acquisition of the Electroencephalogram

Localization 3

Questions: Continue predicting the pattern of EEG deflections induced by the following discharges.

1. See Figure 2-16.

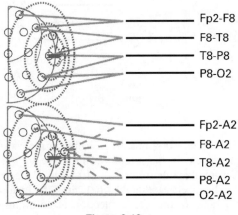

Fp2-F8

F8-T8

T8-P8

P8-O2

Fp2-A2

F8-A2

T8-A2

P8-A2

O2-A2

Figure 2-16.

2. See Figure 2-17.

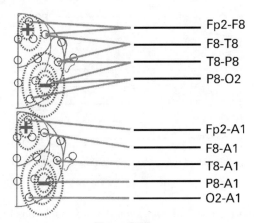

Fp2-F8

F8-T8

T8-P8

P8-O2

Fp2-A1

F8-A1

T8-A1

P8-A1

O2-A1

Figure 2-17.

3. See Figure 2-18.

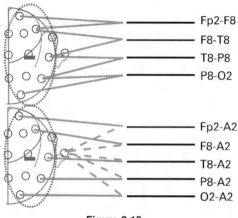

Fp2-F8
F8-T8
T8-P8
P8-O2

Fp2-A2
F8-A2
T8-A2
P8-A2
O2-A2

Figure 2-18.

Answers: 1. This example shows a negative discharge that is isopotential between T8 and A2. Note that phase reversals appear in the referential montage. A *contaminated reference* occurs when the discharge of interest involves the reference electrode. Because channels share a common reference, all channels display the discharge, thereby defeating the localizing abilities and usefulness of the selected referential montage. In this case, selection of an uninvolved reference, such as the contralateral ear, will avoid contamination (Fig. 2-19).

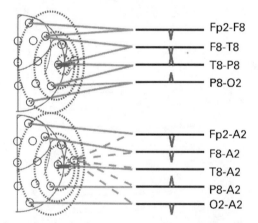

Fp2-F8
F8-T8
T8-P8
P8-O2

Fp2-A2
F8-A2
T8-A2
P8-A2
O2-A2

Figure 2-19. Selection of an uninvolved reference, such as the contralateral ear, will avoid contamination.

2. This example shows the result of a *horizontal dipole*. Only one half of a discharge is usually visible on the upper hemisphere of the scalp recording; the other half of the dipole points down into the inaccessible hemisphere of the scalp model. In some cases, however, dipoles can occur horizontally, thereby exposing both the positive and negative ends of the electrical dipole to regions that are accessible to scalp recordings. In both Figures *A* and *B*, phase reversals are apparent in referential montages. The only time in which phase reversals occur in referential montages are in the case of a contaminated reference or a horizontal dipole (Fig. 2-20).

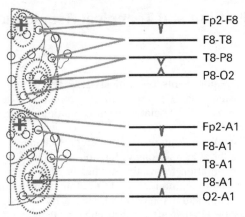

Figure 2-20. Phase reversals occur in referential montages, only in cases of a contaminated reference or a horizontal dipole.

3. This example shows what may occur in a broadly transmitted or a generalized discharge, with a series of unpredictable or isopotential discharges present in bipolar montages. In these cases, the region of highest amplitude on the referential montage identifies the probable source of the discharge (Fig. 2-21).

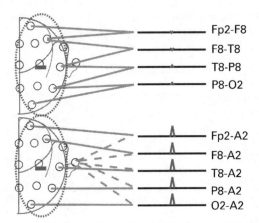

Figure 2-21. The region of highest amplitude on the referential montage identifies the probable source of the discharge.

Clinical Pearls

1. Phase reversals occur in referential montages because of either contaminated references or horizontal dipoles.
2. Focal discharges with a broad field of distribution and generalized discharges are best interpreted with the use of a referential montage.

Calibration and Technical Requirements

The minimal technical requirements of clinical EEG are designed to ensure uniformity in acquisition and to provide a study that is reproducibly interpretable. The American Clinical Neurophysiology Society (née American EEG Society) specifies minimum criteria for routine and neonatal EEG as well as other neurophysiologic tests.

An EEG should consist of a minimum of 16 cerebral channels displayed in at least three montages during the course of the study—a longitudinal bipolar, a transverse bipolar, and a referential montage. The minimum study duration for routine studies is 20 minutes and 1 hour for neonates.

Many requirements are plain common sense. EEG studies must contain name, age, and other identification so that the tracing and its report can be easily linked. Channels and changes to sensitivities and filters must be labeled after every change. Patient movement and state must be commented upon.

Required calibration demonstrates that all channels display EEG voltages as accurately as possible. Calibration consists of three parts: prestudy machine calibration, biocalibration, and post-study machine calibration.

In traditional paper-based systems, machine calibration consists of the application of a calibration signal, usually a 50-μV square wave, into all inputs. The alternating "shark-fin" appearance of the output waveform results from the application of a filter (Fig. 2-22). Machine calibration allows checking whether paper transport is perpendicular to the line of pens, whether pens are aligned, whether pens are equally damped (writing upon the paper with equal force and ease of movement), whether ink flow is smooth, whether filters are applied equally, and whether amplifiers cause equal pen swings for the identical voltage input.

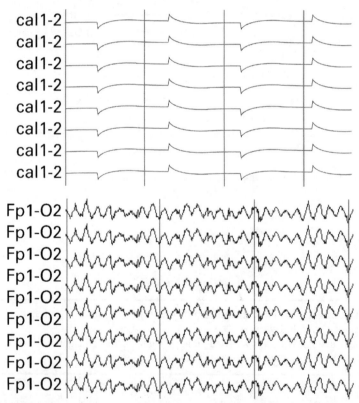

Figure 2-22. During machine calibration (*top*), the alternating "shark-fin" appearance of the output waveform results from the application of a filter. During biocalibration (*bottom*), all channels display the same input from the scalp.

Acquisition of the Electroencephalogram

Biocalibration uses the subject as the signal source, not only double-checking the quality factors mentioned earlier, but also ensuring that the tracing indeed reflects biologically relevant signal. In biocalibration, all channels consist of identical inputs Fp1 to the G1 input and O2 to G2. The montage was designed to amplify biologic signal as much as possible (by virtue of the long interelectrode distance) and to demonstrate the most quickly recognized EEG findings in awake individuals, the posterior waking rhythm, and eye movement artifact.

Finally, a second set of calibrations using the 50-μV calibration signal is performed at the study's end to demonstrate the combinations of filter settings and sensitivities used during the study.

Digital EEG systems vary by manufacturer in the exact method of machine calibration. Some manufacturers dispense with display of calibration and perform calibration internally. For example, at the start of the study, a sinusoidal calibration signal is sent to all amplifiers. The EEG acquisition program reads the output and creates a calibration table that contains a correction factor by which each actual output is multiplied. Each channel is adjusted mathematically to display equal output.

Questions: 1. What is the minimum duration or recording?
2. What montages are required?
3. What channels does standard biocalibration use?

Answers: 1. 20 minutes.
2. Required montages are longitudinal bipolar, transverse bipolar, and one referential.
3. Fp1-O2.

Clinical Pearls

1. Minimum technical criteria for performance of EEGs exist to maintain quality and consistency from lab-to-lab and study-to-study.

2. Although techniques differ by recording method (analog or digital), all EEG studies require machine and biocalibration.

3. Minimum requirements for routine EEG include 16 channels, 3 montages, and 20 minutes duration.

REFERENCE

1. American Electroencephalographic Society: Guideline one: Minimum Technical Requirements for Performing Clinical Electroencephalography. J Clin Neurophysiol 1994; 11:2–5.

The Electro-oculograph (EOG)

Eye leads, once used mainly in polysomnographic studies, are now practical to use in routine EEG recordings. Eye leads can help differentiate anteriorly dominant potentials that originate from eye movement versus cerebral potentials and other noncerebral artifact.

The neural tissue of the retina that lines the globe maintains a negative potential relative to the scalp. The corneal and pupil, however, are positive by virtue of the absence of neurons. Therefore, the anterior portion of the globe is relatively positive to the posterior portion. ''Nerve Negative, Pupil Positive'' is a mnemonic useful in determining the pattern of potentials recorded with eye leads.

Figure 2-23 shows how eye leads channels are created in the examples in this book. Although there are various ways to create eye lead channels, the common feature among them is placement of the paired eye electrodes at opposing elevations—one supraorbital and one infraorbital, with both placed laterally to the eye. This book designates such electrodes as ''E1'' and ''E2''; some labs use ''LOC'' and ''ROC'' for left and right outer canthus.

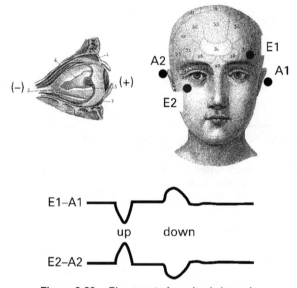

Figure 2-23.   Placement of eye lead channels.

The construction of channels E1-A1 and E2-A2 guarantees that every movement of the eyes will cause a corresponding phase reversal across the two channels. An upward glance causes the left pupil to move toward E1 and record a relative positivity in channel E1-A1. The right pupil simultaneously moves away from E2, and channel E2-A2 records a relative negative potential. Similarly, a downward glance moves the left pupil away from E1 and the right pupil toward E2.

Eye movements, often resembling slow wave activity, sometimes must be differentiated from cerebral anterior activity, without benefit of eye leads in patients who cannot tolerate their application. Even with eye leads, some patients have such continuous and intrusive eye movement that it obscures frontal activities. Technologists in this case may help by recording a portion of the study while holding eyes closed.

Question: The patient in this study was asked to look to either side. To which side did the patient look at point *A* and to which side at *B* in Figure 2-24?

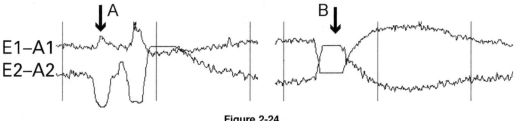

Figure 2-24.

Answer: At *A* the patient looks rightward; at *B*, leftward. As Fig. 2-25 shows, at *A* E1-A1 records upward deflections indicating a negativity, and E2-A2 records downward deflections indicating a positivity. The lateral eye movement that can cause this pattern is a rightward glance as the negative nerve swings toward E2 and the positive pupil toward E1. The opposite occurs at *B*. Note that the high sensitivities used to demonstrate pulse reversal also cause pen blocking.

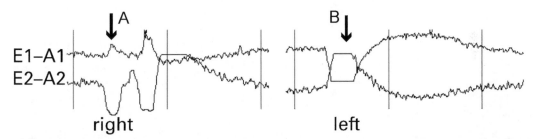

Figure 2-25. *A,* E1-A1 records upward deflections, indicating a negativity, and E2-A2 records downward deflections, indicating a positivity. The lateral eye movement that can cause this pattern is a rightward glance as the negative nerve swings toward E2 and the positive pupil toward E1. *B,* The opposite occurs.

Clinical Pearls

1. The globe is relatively positive anteriorly and negative posteriorly.
2. Eye movement artifact causes phase reversals in properly applied eye electrodes.
3. Eye lead channels can distinguish between potentials that appear on the scalp that arise from eye movement artifact versus potentials of other origins.

Electroencephalographic Description   1

Features of an electroencephalographic (EEG) tracing are described in the following terms:

Frequency. Actual frequency or frequency bands. Some prefer to use units of cycles per second (cps) when referring to biologic activity and units of Hz when referring to nonbiologic activity.

delta	theta	alpha	beta
<4	4– <8	8– <13	≥13

Amplitude. Microvolts (μV) measured from peak to peak. Many refer to low (<25 μV), medium (25–75 μV), and high (>75 μV) voltage amplitudes, but with digital EEG systems it is easier and more precise to refer to the actual amplitude.

Location and distribution. Focal activity is preferentially described in terms of the involved electrodes or in terms of scalp regions. To be accurate, remember that activity over the *temporal region*, for example, refers to the scalp region that is above the temporal lobe and not the temporal lobe itself. More widespread distributions are referred to as *hemispheric* or *generalized* as appropriate.

Symmetry and synchrony. Interhemispheric symmetry indicates that homologous regions from the left and right sides are equal in amplitude. Interhemispheric synchronicity denotes activities that appear simultaneously across left and right hemispheres.

Reactivity. Changes in ongoing activity to endogenous changes in state or to exogenous stimuli are a critical observation in clinical EEG. Certain activities, millimicron (mu) rhythm, for example, are positively identified by specific patterns of reactivity.

Timing. Rhythmicity and its opposite, arhythmicity, require description in many settings. Rhythmicity differs from periodicity in that periodic activities interrupt identifiable background activities interleaved between them, whereas rhythmic activity is continuous.

Morphology. Morphology includes shape (*arciform, epileptiform*), phases (*biphasic, triphasic, polyphasic*), and polarity, which must be noted where appropriate.

Glossaries of accepted terms written by various EEG societies should be consulted in descriptions of EEG findings.

Question: Describe the predominant activity in anterior head regions appearing under the bar in the tracing in Figure 3-1 (see following page).

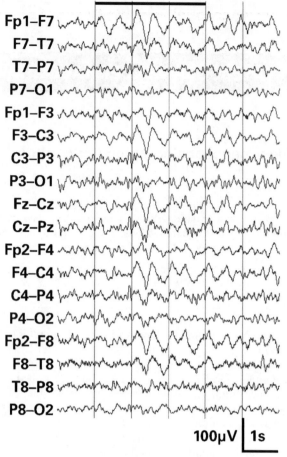

Figure 3-1.

Answer: This is generalized, anteriorly dominant, rhythmic, 2 cps high amplitude delta activity that appears synchronously and symmetrically across each hemisphere. Note that contrary to the composition rules of Strunk and White, long strings of modifiers are encouraged.

REFERENCE

1. Noaschter S, Binnie C, Ebersole J: Glossary of terms most commonly used by clinical electroencephalographers and proposal for the report form for the EEG findings. Electroencephalogr Clin Neurophysiol 1999; 5(Suppl 2): 21–512.

Electroencephalographic Description   2

Electroencephalographers refer to three seemingly simple concepts in ways that seem confusing to those new to EEG: background versus foreground, rhythmicity versus periodicity, evolution versus stationary.

Background activity. Any "activity representing the setting in which a given normal or abnormal pattern appears and from which such pattern is distinguished." In other words, background activity is any ongoing activity upon which something of interest in the foreground requires description. Background activity is not a shorthand term for "the gist of the recording."

Rhythm. Any continuously repeating waveform with a constant or near constant period. Rhythmic activity occurs continuously; each waveform is followed by a similar waveform and is not interrupted by dissimilar activity.

Periodic activity. Any waveform or complex of waveforms that repeats at a more-or-less regular rate. Unlike rhythmic activity, periodic activity occurs upon ongoing, dissimilar activities. EEG activities of cerebral origin seldom occur with metronymic periodicity. Such regular timing implies artifact. Instead, cerebral periodic discharges usually occur in a quasi-periodic pattern, in which each complex is separated by a range of durations.

Arrhythmic activity. Any pattern with inconstant, irregular period. The term *polymorphic* is used synonymously for *arrhythmic* by many, but others reserve *polymorphic* to describe irregularly shaped activity rather than irregularly timed activity. In many cases, the distinction is small because both properties are usually present in these patterns.

Evolution. Gradual changes in amplitude, frequency, or spatial distribution of rhythms (Fig. 3-2). It is a characteristic of ictal discharges to evolve in a stereotypic fashion as the discharge continues, whereas nonictal activity, whether rhythmic or periodic, tends to remain constant at different stages of its appearance.

nonevolving periodic transients on theta background activity (EKG artifact)

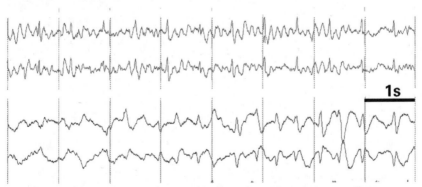

evolving rhythmic sharp wave discharges on delta frequency background activity (neonatal seizure)

Figure 3-2.   Evolution refers to gradual changes in amplitude, frequency, or spatial distribution of rhythms.

Question: Match patterns *(A)*, *(B)*, and *(C)* in Figure 3-3 with the terms *rhythmic, quasi-periodic*, and *arrhythmic*.

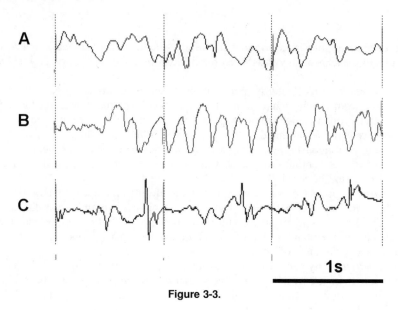

Figure 3-3.

Answer: *(A)* arrhythmic activity, *(B)* rhythmic activity, *(C)* quasi-periodic activity

REFERENCE

1. Noaschter S, Binnie C, Ebersole J: Glossary of terms most commonly used by clinical electroencephalographers and proposal for the report form for the EEG findings. Electroencephalogr Clin Neurophysiol 1999; 5(Suppl 2): 21–512.

Interictal Epileptiform Discharges

An important finding in EEG is the *interictal epileptiform discharge* (IED). A necessary skill in the interpretation of the EEG is the visual detection of IEDs and their distinction from discharges that are benign or are the result of artifact. The task requires a clear understanding of the terminology of IEDs. The following terminology is from the general to the specific:

Transient. The general term for any brief potential encountered in a tracing.

Sharp transient. Any transient potential with an *epileptiform* (sharp) morphology (Fig. 3-4). Note that *epileptiform* is synonymous with sharp and is a morphologic descriptor rather than a clinical predictor. All epileptiform discharges are not associated with epileptic seizures, and a sharp transient may or may not have clinical significance.

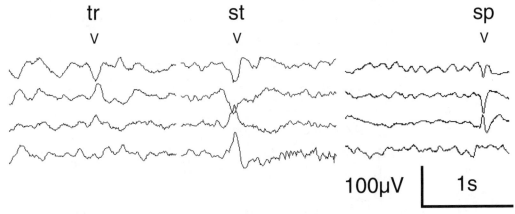

Figure 3-4. Examples of a transient (tr), sharp transient (st), and spike (sp) discharges.

More specific terms carry clinical significance.

Sharp wave. Any sharp transient that interrupts and stands out from ongoing background activity, has a sharp component with a duration measured at its base between 70–200 ms, is often followed by an aftercoming slow wave potential, and is not attributable to artifact. If these criteria are met, then the potential in question can be termed a *sharp wave,* a finding that carries the significance of association with epileptic seizures. In most cases, the sharp component and aftercoming slow wave have a surface-negative potential, an important property to observe because many surface-positive discharges indicate a benign, normal origin.

Spike. A sharp transient that meets the criteria for sharp waves, except that duration of the sharp component is briefer (between 20 and 70 ms) than that of a sharp wave. Beyond duration, there is little difference between the two. Spikes and sharp waves are both referred to as IEDs, and both are associated with a susceptibility to recurrent epileptic seizures. Some authorities refer to IEDs as *epileptogenic.* Although perhaps a misnomer (because IEDs are not the cause of epilepsy, merely the result), epileptogenic in the common sense refers to the association between IEDs and epilepsy.

Sometimes a sharp transient cannot be identified either as an artifact, a clearly benign finding, or as a definite IED. In this case, the clinical significance of the sharp transient is unclear. The previously described hierarchy reflects that interpretation of transients follows an algorithm. Once a sharp transient is encountered, one must decide whether it is of cerebral or noncerebral origin. If cerebral in origin, it must be classified as a normal finding, a benign variant, or a clinically significant IED.

Question: Provide the best term to define the discharges shown at *(A)* and at *(B)* in Figure 3-5.

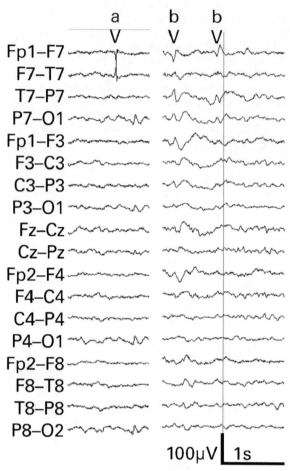

Figure 3-5.

Answer: *(A)* = transient (electrode pop), *(B)* = spike. At *(A)*, the transient is a brief (<20 ms) biphasic, extremely sharp discharge confined to a single electrode, F7. An *electrode pop* artifact results from abrupt release of current from an electrode that has developed a capacitative charge. In *(B)*, there are two spike discharges that are isopotential between F7-T7 corresponding to the anterior midtemporal region. These negative potential discharges interrupt and stand out from background activity, have durations between 20–70 ms, are followed by a negative slow potential, and cannot be explained as an artifact.

Clinical Pearls

1.   A sharp transient is a descriptive term denoting any transient potential that is sharply contoured.

2.   Spikes and sharp waves are discharges that interrupt background activity, have a cerebral potential field, are usually followed by an after potential with the same polarity, and have durations ranging from 20–70 ms (spikes) and 70–200 ms (sharp waves).

3.   Sharp transients must be classified as having or lacking a cerebral origin, and if originating from the brain, must be further classified as *normal,* a *benign epileptiform variant,* or as an *IED.*

4.   Spikes and sharp waves (IEDs) have a strong association with epileptic seizures and are often termed *epileptogenic.*

PATIENT 1

A 55-year-old woman with recurrent sharp transients

An EKG is requested to evaluate possible interictal epileptiform discharges status post head trauma and unspecified seizures. The tracing was recorded with the patient awake. She is taking phenytoin.

Question: Explain the origin of the periodic sharp discharges in this ipsilateral-ear referential montage.

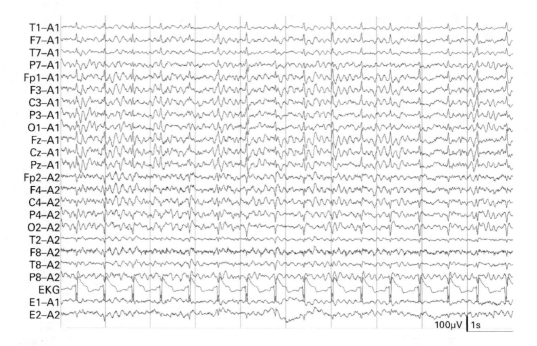

Answer: Periodic sharp transients arise from EKG artifact. The direction of the QRS complex is *up* (negative) in channels referenced to the left ear and *down* (positive) in those referenced to the right because of the orientation of cerebral leads in relation to the axis of the QRS cardiac complex.

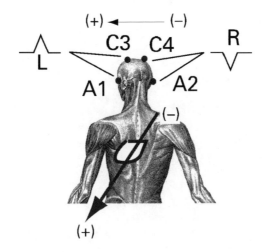

Discussion: Whereas the brain generates signals in the microvolt range, the heart generates signals with amplitudes in the millivolt range, about a three-magnitude difference. EKG artifact, therefore, is a common finding in many routine tracings.

Fortunately, the abilities of modern EEG equipment facilitate the distinction between EKG artifact and cerebral activity. Most laboratories acquire EKG by using two chest leads and display EKG as one channel within most montages. The QRS complex shows the vector of the depolarization of the ventricles. The ventricles depolarize from apex to the ventricular base, causing a wave of relatively positive potential. Depending on the cardiac axis of an individual patient, the electrical axis of the QRS complex is usually not aligned with the vertical axis of the patient and forms a skewed vector.

In this example, channels referenced to A1 have an upward pointing EKG deflection because the EKG potential is more negative among the cerebral channels that are rightward of the left ear. Channels referenced to A2 have downward pointing EKG artifact because the cerebral channels, leftward of the right ear, register an EKG positivity relative to the right ear.

Because of long interelectrode distances, referential montages are particularly susceptible to EKG artifact. Patients with relatively short necks, such as infants or football linemen (one and the same in the opinion of some), are particularly apt to show EKG artifact, especially in montages constructed from ear references because of their relative proximity to the heart. Technicians can try to correct EKG artifact by repositioning of the head to bring the electrical vector of the head in line with the cardiac vector. A *balanced reference* obtained by adjusting the impedance of ear references until EKG cancels out is another method of minimizing EKG artifact.

Occasionally, the EKG channel can serve a greater purpose than one of mere artifact detection. Cardiac dysrhythmias can be identified and even correlated with clinical symptoms if they occur during the tracing.

Clinical Pearls

1. EKG artifact can superimpose itself on normal activity; care in interpretations of IEDs must rule out EKG artifact.
2. Referential montages are the most susceptible to EKG artifact.
3. EEGs should be supplemented by an EKG channel to facilitate the distinction between EKG artifact and cerebral potentials.

PATIENT 2

A 20-year-old man with headaches

A 20-year-old man is evaluated for headaches that involves a feeling of dissociation during their worst presentation and are thought to be seizures by his primary physician. He takes no medications. The patient was awake during the tracing below. He did not have any spells during the tracing.

Question: What normal waking activity is represented by the tracing?

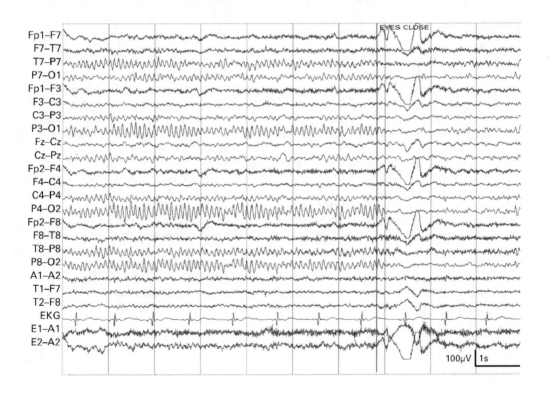

Answer: 10 cps, posteriorly dominant, symmetric, well-regulated alpha rhythm that attenuates with eye opening.

Discussion: Interpretation of the electroencephalogram (EEG) starts with evaluation of the posterior waking rhythm, or *alpha rhythm.* Whereas alpha activity simply describes a frequency band, alpha rhythm denotes a pattern of EEG findings that, in the awake patient, is the main herald of a normal tracing. A normal alpha rhythm has the following characteristics:

State-dependence. Alpha rhythm is seen during quiet wakefulness. Agitated, awake individuals may not display an alpha rhythm. Because intense concentration (as when performing mental arithmetic) can block alpha rhythm, it may be absent in some preoccupied, and not necessarily agitated subjects. An alpha rhythm may not be explicitly demonstrable in restless children until right before falling asleep. Patients who are persistently drowsy despite attempts at waking may also not show an alpha rhythm. In these cases, an absence of alpha rhythm, lacking other indications, is not an abnormality. On the other hand, the alpha rhythm (or its variants) is an obligate finding in normal, relaxed, developmentally appropriate people.

Frequency. The frequency of alpha rhythm in adults ranges from >8 to 13 cps, with a mean frequency of 10 cps. Although a frequency of 8 cps can be present in a normal adult, it is more likely the result of borderline encephalopathy. Adults should maintain the same frequency from study to study, with a drop of >1 cps suggesting pathology. Drowsiness and medications can also cause slowing of the alpha rhythm in an otherwise normal person.

Amplitude. The voltage of the adult alpha rhythm recorded from the scalp ranges from 15–50μV. No pathology is associated with higher voltages.

Location. The alpha rhythm is maximally present in the occipital channels.

Symmetry. The voltage of alpha rhythm recorded from the right hemisphere is often slightly higher than that recorded from the left, usually not more than 20%. The asymmetry does not arise from brain activity; instead, differences in the underlying bone thickness, probably due to the torcula (the confluence of the transverse and sagittal sinuses), influence the impedance and thus the voltage of the alpha rhythm recorded from either hemisphere. Asymmetry of alpha rhythm exceeding 50% is abnormal, but its interpretation as abnormal should be cautiously entertained if asymmetry is the only abnormality. Problems with electrodes, such as impedance asymmetry or misplacement of electrodes, are the most likely culprits in cases of isolated voltage asymmetry of alpha rhythm.

Morphology. Regulation denotes a regularity of morphology. A well-regulated alpha rhythm approaches a sinusoidal, monomorphic waveform with little variation throughout the tracing. Alpha rhythm often appears in long, spindle-shaped runs. Spindling is thought to arise from the differing signal generators of the alpha rhythm, each with slightly varying frequencies and amplitudes. Patterns of reinforcement and interference result when these separate waveforms combine.

Reactivity. Eye opening attenuates alpha rhythm. This distinguishes alpha rhythm from other activities—normal and abnormal—sharing the alpha frequency band. Its demonstration by the EEG technician is an obligate procedure during performance of the tracing. Patients unable to cooperate with voluntary eye opening and closure should have eyes passively closed and opened at some point.

In this particular patient with headaches and feelings of dissociation, the requesting physician was interested in the possibility that dissociation may represent seizures. Although this tracing lacked evidence of interictal epileptiform abnormalities, some subjects with epilepsy have normal interictal EEGs.

The Normal Waking Electroencephalogram

Clinical Pearls

1. The normal, relaxed waking EEG should contain an example of alpha rhythm or one of its variants.

2. Alpha rhythm has characteristic frequency, location, symmetry, and reactivity that must be demonstrated on the record to distinguish it from other alpha frequency activities.

3. The normal adult alpha rhythm frequency ranges from >8–13 cps with a mean of 10 cps.

REFERENCES

1. Bancaud J, Hecaen H, Lairy GC: Modifications de la reactivitie EEG, troubles de fonctions symboliques et troubles confusionnels dans les lesions hemispherics localisees. Electroencephalogr Clin Neurophysiol 1955; 7:295–302.
2. Kellaway P: Orderly approach to visual analysis: Characteristics of the normal EEG in children and adults. In Daly DD, Pedley TA (eds): Current Practice of Clinical Electroencephalography. New York, Raven, pp 139–199.
3. Petersen I, Eeg-Olofsson O: The development of the EEG in normal children from the age of 1 to 15 years: Nonparoxysmal activity. Neuropadiatrie 1971; 2:247–304.

PATIENT 3

A 12-month-old boy with staring spells

A 12-month-old boy has frequent staring spells. He has normal developmental milestones and takes no medications.

The tracing below was recorded with the patient awake.

Questions: What is the frequency of the alpha rhythm? Is it appropriate for the patient's age?

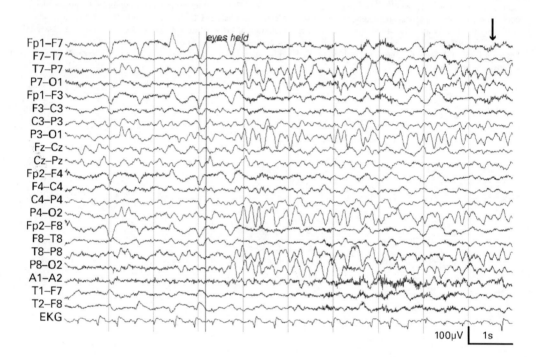

Answers: 6 cps alpha rhythm, best seen at the last part of the sample *(arrow)*. This frequency is appropriate for the patient's age.

Discussion: A waking posterior rhythm becomes evident in most infants by age 3 months and is sometimes discernible earlier. The frequency of alpha rhythm increases with maturation, generally attaining the adult lower limit of >8 cps by age 3.

Many studies have determined the normal frequency for age. The plot shown below is a composite of three references. The two older studies show upper and lower limits of a cohort of normal children, most studied longitudinally. The more recent study shows the upper and lower 95% confidence limits of frequencies of normal children. Note that the increase in frequency is rapid through the first year of life and gradually slows thereafter.

No pathologic conditions are associated with alpha rhythm frequencies that are faster than the normal range, although care should be taken that the observed supranormal frequencies are the posterior waking rhythm.

Frequencies slower than the 95% confidence interval, if drowsy state is excluded, should be considered an indicator of a nonspecific encephalopathy.

Determining the frequency of alpha rhythm in infants and small children can be difficult because, when fully awake, they often maintain eye opening and block alpha rhythm, leaving behind other activities that can mistakenly be counted as alpha rhythm. Furthermore, when alpha rhythm can usually be best seen in these young subjects—quietly restful with eyes closed to elicit a and approaching sleep—the alpha rhythm can be slowed from drowsiness. The solution is to have the EEG technologist hold the eyes closed to elicit a sample of waking alpha rhythm.

Also adding to the difficulty is that, in children, occipital slow wave discharges are often normally superimposed upon faster occipital frequencies, as seen in this case. The lower limit of Lindsey's study of the longitudinal development of the posterior rhythm probably reflects this intermixing of posterior slow waves with the best "alpha rhythm" frequency. Current technique is to count the best frequency of the posterior rhythm, as reflected in Smith's study of alpha rhythm development.

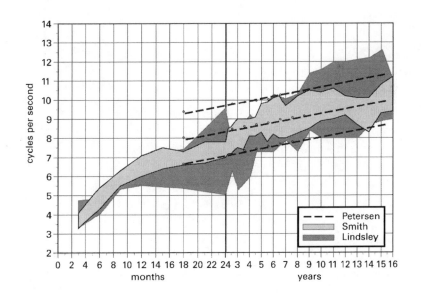

The Normal Waking Electroencephalogram

51

Clinical Pearls

1. Alpha rhythm is first seen at age 3 months and increases with maturation.
2. Alpha rhythm frequency of >8 cps is attained around age 3.
3. Explicit demonstration of alpha rhythm in children is required in most studies of those too young to cooperate with instructions.

REFERENCES

1. Eeg-Olofsson O, Petersen I: The development of the EEG in normal children from the age of 1 to 15 years: Paroxysmal activity. Neuropadiatrie 1971; 4:375–404.
2. Lindsley DB: Longitudinal study of the occipital alpha rhythm in normal children: Frequency amplitude standards. J Genet Psychol 1939; 55:197–213.
3. Smith JR: The electroencephalograph during normal infancy childhood. I: Rhythmic activities present in the neonate and their subsequent development. J Genet Psychol 1938; 53:431–453.

PATIENT 4

A 6-year-old girl with seizures after a urinary tract infection

A 6-year-old girl, seizure-free for 3 years, is evaluated after recurrence of generalized tonic-clonic seizures during a severe urinary tract infection. She takes topiramate and felbamate.

The tracing below was recorded with the patient awake.

Question: Is the posterior rhythm normal for age? Note the transverse longitudinal montage.

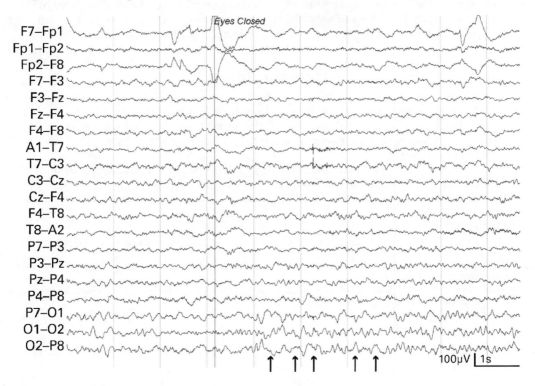

Answer: Sporadic delta activity *(arrows)* accompanies posterior alpha activity in the 10–10.5 cps range and appears with eye closure. Posterior slow waves of youth are an age-dependent normal finding. The alpha rhythm is normal for age.

Discussion: One difficulty the waking EEG of a child presents is the accurate distinction between normal and abnormal occipital delta activity. *Posterior slow waves of youth* are most likely to occur in children between ages 8 and 14 and are rare beyond age 21.

Posterior slow waves of youth present as polyphasic, sporadic, or arrhythmic occipital delta activities that otherwise behave like the alpha rhythm. They appear maximally during relaxed wakefulness and disappear with drowsiness or sleep. Like alpha rhythm, posterior slow waves of youth are frequently higher in amplitude on the right side. Alpha rhythm in the alpha frequency band is typically superimposed upon the higher amplitude slow wave discharges, giving the occipital alpha rhythm a poorly regulated appearance. Most importantly, similar to alpha rhythm, posterior slow waves of youth attenuate with eye opening.

In distinction to posterior slow waves of youth, unreactive or rhythmic delta activity that interrupts alpha rhythm is abnormal.

Clinical Pearls

1. Posterior low waves of youth are a frequent finding in normal children.

2. Posterior slow waves of youth are distinguished from abnormal slowing in that they are present with age-appropriate alpha rhythm and, like alpha rhythm, attenuate with eye opening.

3. Reports of abnormal posterior slowing in children should be greeted with skepticism if reactivity, state, and other posterior activities are not adequately described.

REFERENCES

1. Aird RB, Gastaut Y: Occipital posterior electroencephalographic rhythms. Electroencephalogr Clin Neurophysiol 1959; 11:637–656.
2. Eeg-Olofsson O, Petersen I: The development of the EEG in normal children from the age of 1 to 15 years: Paroxysmal activity. Neuropadiatrie 1971; 4:375–404.
3. Petersen I, Eeg-Olofsson O: The development of the EEG in normal children from the age of 1 to 15 years: Nonparoxysmal activity. Neuropadiatrie 1971; 2:247–304.

PATIENT 5

A 40-year-old man with depression

A 40-year-old man presents with medically intractable depression before electroconvulsive therapy (ECT). Medications are Zoloft and valproic acid.

Question: What frequency is the alpha rhythm? Is it best counted at sample *A* or sample *B?*

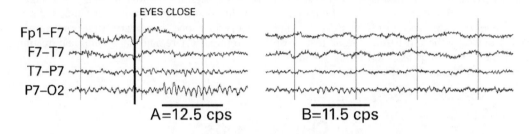

Answer: 11.5 cps, sample *B*. Sample *A* shows a transiently increased frequency of approximately 12.5 cps after eye closure, called *squeak phenomenon*.

Discussion: The frequency of the alpha rhythm may not be stable throughout a single study. Its frequency can be increased immediately after eye closure. For example, in the tracing the alpha frequency immediately after eye closure artifact at sample *A* is approximately 12 cps, whereas later in the recording at sample *B* it is more accurately counted at 11.5 cps. This transient increase in the frequency of alpha rhythm immediately after eye closure is called *squeak phenomenon*, after the brief harsh squeaking sound made by the old EEG systems that arose from the sound of pens "squeaking" with the abrupt onset of activity after eye closure.

Drowsiness is a state that commonly decreases the frequency of the alpha rhythm. For accuracy's sake, alpha rhythm should be counted during maximum alertness but not limited to intervals immediately after eye closure. Given these limitations, alpha rhythm should be assigned the highest frequency not increased by squeak phenomenon.

In this patient, the alpha rhythm outside of squeak phenomenon was normal. This suggests that his depression is a primary mood disorder rather than one secondary to encephalopathy. Therefore, ECT remains an appropriate treatment.

Clinical Pearls

1. Squeak phenomenon is a transient increase in alpha frequency following eye closure that may cause overestimation of alpha rhythm.

2. Drowsiness can decrease the frequency of alpha rhythm.

3. The "true" alpha rhythm frequency is the fastest frequency during maximum arousal from samples not limited to those immediately after eye closure.

The Normal Waking Electroencephalogram

PATIENT 6

A 25-year-old man with spells of loss of consciousness

A 25-year-old man is evaluated for recent onset of spells of loss of consciousness and wandering. He is on no medications.

The tracing below was recorded with the patient awake.

Question: Is the posterior rhythm before eye opening (EO) normal?

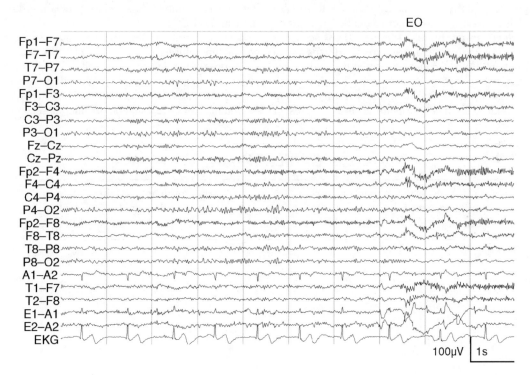

Answer: Yes. Approximately 20 cps posterior rhythm admixed with 10 cps posterior rhythm is an example of fast alpha rhythm variant, a normal finding.

Discussion: In some recordings, the 8–13 cps frequency of the alpha rhythm is infrequent, even in relaxed, normal subjects. Instead, the majority of the posterior waking rhythm consists of low amplitude (<25 µV) activities in the beta frequency band, usually at a frequency double that of a more typical alpha rhythm frequency. Sometimes the faster, harmonic frequency overlies that of the slower, alpha frequency activity, giving a poorly regulated appearance to the occipital activity. This pattern is called *fast alpha rhythm variant*. In this example, 20 cps activities interrupt or overlie more typical 10 cps alpha rhythm. Both frequencies attenuate with eye opening.

Like alpha rhythm, fast alpha rhythm variant attenuates with eye opening and is present during the same state of relaxed wakefulness. Fast alpha rhythm variant is normal. Strict interpretation requires that brief bursts of alpha rhythm in the alpha frequency band at an integer multiple of the posterior fast frequency be present. Sometimes, however, the sole finding is of low-amplitude fast activities. Occasionally, in such "reluctant" individuals, a search for alpha frequency activities may be successful only during hyperventilation (a standard procedure during routine EEG).

Because events of loss of consciousness were not captured during this routine EEG, this normal study does not rule out the possibility that these events are epileptic in etiology. We will discuss in subsequent cases the specificity and sensitivity of the routine EEG in evaluation of epileptic seizures.

Clinical Pearl

Fast alpha rhythm variant appears as a posteriorly dominant, symmetric, low-amplitude beta frequency activity—typically double the fundamental alpha rhythm frequency—that attenuates with eye opening.

PATIENT 7

A 21-year-old man with new-onset seizures

The patient had a closed head injury 6 months before the tracing and now has generalized tonic-clonic seizures. His only medication is phenytoin.

The technician noted a lack of scalp abnormalities. The patient is awake.

Questions: Does this tracing show significant asymmetry of alpha rhythm in sample *A*? What does the improved symmetry in sample *B* suggest as to the source of asymmetry in sample *A*?

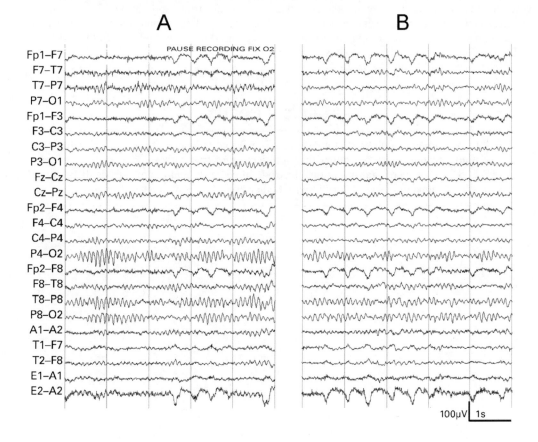

Answers: The amplitude of alpha rhythm on the left side during sample *A* is <50% that of the right, a significant asymmetry. Impedance mismatch, electrode misplacement, scalp asymmetry, and head placement can all contribute to asymmetry of the alpha rhythm.

Discussion: The voltage across any two points is proportional to impedance. *Impedance mismatch* of one electrode relative to others can artifactually enhance the amplitude of the voltage measured from the electrode pair that contains the ''bad'' electrode.

Misplacement of an electrode can also increase apparent voltage, because an increased distance between the electrode pair also increases the impedance. In this case, the increase in interelectrode distances between O2 and its pairs leads to an artifactual amplification of the alpha rhythm on that side.

The condition of the scalp can affect symmetry. The technician should note the presence of scalp edema, old scarring, cranial malformation, or any other patient factors that can contribute to differences in electrical properties of scalp regions.

Head placement should be noted, if alpha rhythm amplitude is variable during the tracing. Increased pressure on the electrode can induce transiently decreased impedance.

In this example, after the pause in the recording, when the technologist corrected placement of the O2 electrode and checked its impedance, the amplitude of the alpha rhythm on the right side decreased to normal relative to the left.

Clinical Pearls

1. Asymmetry of alpha rhythm, especially without evidence of other abnormalities, is often a technical artifact rather than a reflection of true pathology.

2. Scalp edema or malformation, electrode impedance, and interelectrode distances must be evaluated before determining whether amplitude asymmetry is abnormal.

PATIENT 8

A 36-year-old woman with depression and spells

A 36-year-old woman has spells of altered consciousness exacerbated by stress. Medications are fluoxetine and carbamazepine.

Questions: What is the alpha rhythm frequency under the bar in this ipsilateral ear-referential montage? Is it in the normal range?

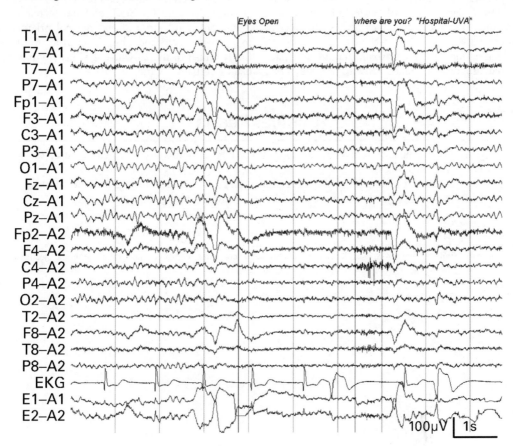

Answers: 7 cps, an abnormally slow alpha rhythm.

Discussion: An alpha rhythm that fulfills all of the other criteria of alpha rhythm, except for a too slow frequency, is commonly called a *slow alpha rhythm.* Some authorities suggest that the term *slow posterior waking rhythm* be used to avoid a contradiction of terms between "alpha rhythm" and the presence of theta activity.

Slowing of the alpha rhythm can be caused by both normal and pathologic conditions.

Insufficient alerting: Persistent drowsiness can be present, especially in sleep-deprived patients. In these cases, the EEG technician should document the means and results of attempts at arousal.

Medication effects: Carbamazepine and phenytoin are apt to induce slowing of the alpha rhythm regardless of whether blood serum levels exceed the therapeutic range. Other medications with central nervous system effects can also cause slowing of alpha rhythm—usually along with other EEG abnormalities—when present in toxic or near-toxic levels.

Nonspecific borderline or mild encephalopathy: Mild metabolic or toxic abnormalities or static encephalopathy can cause slowing of the alpha rhythm.

In the current case, there were no other abnormalities in the EEG, and the technologist documented full arousal and normal orientation to person, place, and time. Therefore, the most likely cause of the slowing of alpha rhythm was use of carbamazepine.

Clinical Pearls

1. Slow alpha rhythm is the result of mild encephalopathy, medication use, or persistent drowsiness.

2. Sufficient testing from the technologist and accurate accounting of medications from requesting physicians are required to distinguish among these choices.

REFERENCE

1. Duncan JS, Smith SJ, Forster A, et al: Effects of the removal of phenytoin, carbamazepine, valproate on the electroencephalogram. Epilepsia 1989; 30(5):590–596.

PATIENT 9

A 16-year-old boy with possible absence seizures

A 16-year-old boy has staring spells in school. Sertraline is his only medication.
The tracing below was recorded with the patient awake.

Question: What is the name of the rhythm present in the left centroparietal region? Describe it.

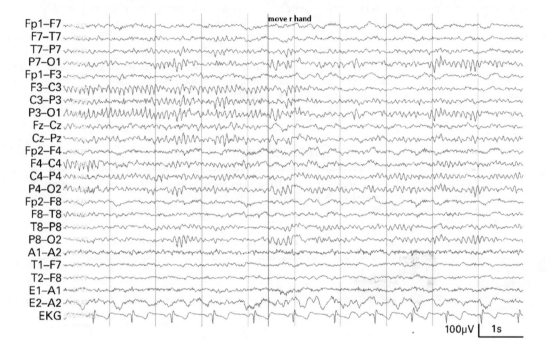

Answer: Rhythmic, 11 cps, arc-shaped activity appears during wakefulness and attenuates with movement of the contralateral hand. This is an example of *mu rhythm*.

Discussion: Mu rhythm is the endogenous activity of the awake sensorimotor cortex. Unlike alpha rhythm, its presence may be difficult to establish, and its absence is not abnormal in a routine tracing. Mu rhythm is present in 10–15% of waking tracings. Frequently it may be difficult to see because it may be masked by a higher-amplitude or anteriorly displaced alpha rhythm. It must be distinguished from the alpha rhythm so that the frequency of the alpha rhythm is not overestimated.

Location. Central parasagittal regions and frequently seen on one side only.

Frequency. In the alpha range, typically 10–11 cps.

Amplitude. Typically near or below the amplitude of the alpha rhythm. Because the skull both dampens EEG amplitude and acts as a high-frequency filter, the mu rhythm can be usually high in amplitude and appear especially sharp in morphology over regions with a focal skull defect. Breach rhythm originally referred to the phenomenon of enhanced mu rhythm in skull defects.

Morphology. Mu rhythm received its name from its resemblance to the Greek letter μ, with waveforms occurring in series of joined arcs.

Reactivity. The key in demonstration of mu rhythm, and its differentiation from alpha rhythm, is that mu rhythm attenuates with movement of the contralateral hand. Even thinking of moving the hand will attenuate mu rhythm.

Clinical Pearls

1. Mu rhythm consists of arc-shaped, 10–11 cps parasagittal rhythmic activities that attenuate with contralateral limb movement.

2. Mistaking mu rhythm for alpha rhythm can cause miscounting of the alpha rhythm frequency.

3. Mu rhythm can be artifactually enhanced by underlying skull defects.

REFERENCE

1. Cobb WA, Guiloff RJ, Cast J: Breach rhythm: The EEG related to skull defects. Electroencephalogr Clin Neurophysiol 1979; 47:251–271.

PATIENT 10

A 17-year-old boy with autism and episodic rage attacks

A 17-year-old autistic boy presents for evaluation of episodes of rage thought to be consistent with epileptic seizures. The study is performed during sedation because of violent behavior and a failure of a previous attempt at an unsedated study.

The tracing below was recorded with the patient sedated and unresponsive. Medications during the study were single dose of midazolam (administered 2 hours before the study) and an ongoing low-dose propofol intravenous drip. That was gradually decreased during the study.

Questions: Are the beta activities in the sample normal? Does the ongoing sedation decrease the useful information of the tracing?

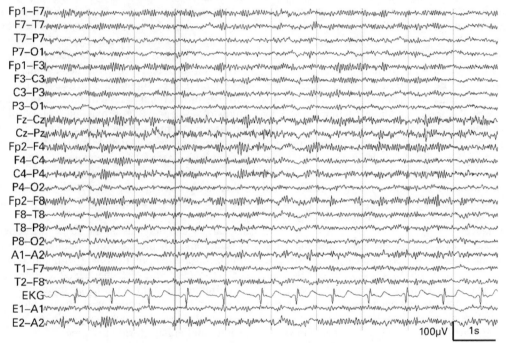

Answers: The tracing shows diffusely distributed, symmetric beta activity from 19–22 cps, with voltages exceeding 25 µV. Beta activity with these properties is commonly called *enhanced beta activity* and is due to effects of medication. Sedation may decrease the sensitivity of the study to determine degree of encephalopathy and the occurrence of the spells in question.

Discussion: Beta activity is often encountered in EEG recordings but varies in significance, depending on its characteristics.

Frequency. Frequencies above 13 cps comprise the beta frequency band and are often referred to as *fast frequencies.* Activity that exceeds 25 cps may be difficult to discern from muscle artifact when recording from the scalp. Conversely, the scalp and skull act as effective high-frequency filters, as they remove the preponderance of fast frequencies that can be recorded faithfully through electrocorticography.

Amplitude. In most subjects, beta activity is not a prominent feature. Beta activity remains less than 10 µV in 70% of subjects and less than 25 µV in 98% of healthy subjects. Its amplitude is symmetric across each hemisphere.

Location. Beta activity appears more frequently in anterior channels due to the prominence of the posterior alpha rhythm in waking recordings.

The most common abnormality that involves beta activity is an exaggeration in amplitude. Beta activity with amplitude exceeding 25 µV for the majority of the study is commonly called *enhanced beta activity.* Enhanced beta activity arises in both pathologic and nonpathologic circumstances.

Sedative-hypnotic medications are the most frequent cause of diffuse enhancement of beta activities within the 18–25 cps range. Barbiturates and benzodiazepines are historically the most frequently cited, but most sedative-hypnotics and many antidepressants may enhance beta activity when used in clinically relevant dosages. In the case of this patient, drug ingestion was clearly documented. Its presence in a patient taking no admitted medications, however, suggests that sedative-hypnotics have been ingested. In polysomnography, enhanced beta activity may appear as *pseudospindles* and, by mimicking sleep spindles, may confound proper identification of stage 2 sleep.

Sleep-wake state can affect the relative predominance of beta activity. Light drowsiness may transiently and diffusely enhance beta activity.

Focal skull defects often lead to focal enhancement of the relative amount and amplitude of fast activity, often called *breach rhythm.*

Focal tumors or cortical dysplasias may be associated with focal enhancement of fast frequencies, a rarer, unexpected finding in the age of modern neuroimaging.

Sedation during EEG is problematic for three reasons.

First, medications can affect the EEG; that is, changes induced by sedation, such as diffuse slowing of the predominant frequency, can be identical to those associated with encephalopathy.

Second, different sedative medications may have facilitive or suppressive effects on the occurrence of interictal or ictal discharges in certain kinds of epilepsies. For example, propofol is thought by some to ''activate'' (facilitate the appearance of) interictal epileptiform discharges, a seemingly paradoxical tendency, despite its usefulness in the treatment of status epilepticus. Other medications, such as benzodiazepines, often suppress interictal epileptiform activity. Suppression or activation of interictal epileptiform discharges also depends on the suspected epilepsy syndrome. In the case of childhood absence epilepsy, for example, treatment with anticonvulsants can obliterate the characteristic abnormal EEG findings. On the other hand, treatment with anticonvulsants typically used in symptomatic partial epilepsies does not change the occurrence of interictal epileptiform discharges.

Third, current practice discourages ''conscious sedation'' in laboratories unless there is adequate monitoring of vital signs and availability of appropriately trained staff in resuscitation.

In this particular case, no abnormalities beyond enhanced beta activity during sedation were seen. The patient was later managed with behavioral modification strategies and mood-stabilizing agents.

Clinical Pearls

1. Low-amplitude, symmetric beta activity is part of the normal waking EEG.

2. Diffuse beta activity >25 μV for the majority of a routine study is evidence of abnormal enhancement.

3. Enhancement of beta activity must be interpreted in context of state: beta activity can also be enhanced due to drowsiness.

4. Sedation during EEG must be undertaken with the proper safety precautions. Sedation can limit the information available from the study.

REFERENCES

1. Eeg-Olofsson O: The development of the EEG in normal adolescents from the age of 16 to 21 years. Neuropadiatrie 1971; 3:11–45.
2. Gotman J, Koffler D: Interictal spiking increases after seizures but does not after decreases in medication. Electroencephalogr Clin Neurophysiol 1989; 72:7–15.
3. Hodkinson BP, Frith RW, Mee EW: Propofol the electroencephalogram. Lancet 1987; 2(8574):1518.
4. Petersen I, Eeg-Olofsson O: The development of the EEG in normal children from the age of 1 to 15 years: Nonparoxysmal activity. Neuropadiatrie 1971; 2:247–304.

PATIENT 11

A 14-year-old boy with head trauma and episodic rage attacks

A 14-year-old boy presents for evaluation of episodic rage following a motor vehicle accident, resulting in skull fracture and trauma to the right centroparietal region. Medications are clonidine and fluoxetine.

The study was performed during poorly cooperative wakefulness.

Questions: Are the fast frequencies shown in the tracing normal? Do they indicate sedative-hypnotic use?

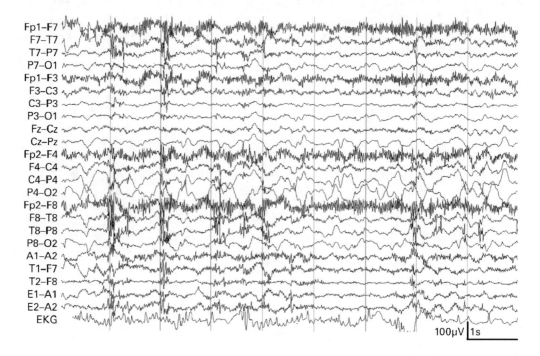

Answers: The tracing shows symmetric beta activities in the 20–35 cps range in anterior channels that arise from frontalis muscle artifact. Periodic bursts of diffuse beta activities mark chewing artifact. Frequent delta activities and distortion of electrocardiogram (EKG) signal originate from patient movement. These artifacts, if present during the entire tracing, limit the ability to interpret the recording, are not of cerebral origin, and do not indicate sedative-hypnotic use.

Discussion: Electromyographic (EMG) activity occupies the beta frequency band. When recorded from the scalp, activities above approximately 25 cps are difficult to discern from muscle activity. Central channels are usually spared because of the relative lack of underlying muscle, but frontalis, temporalis, and masseter muscle activity can render EEG illegible if continuous.

Technologists can improve muscle artifact in cooperative patients by asking the patient to open their mouths, thereby relaxing most scalp musculature. Sleep, either spontaneous or induced by sedation, may be necessary for the uncooperative.

Standard recommendations for the format and content of the standard EEG report are given in the below reference. In addition, many recommend that the clinical interpretation include one of four basic conclusions: (1) normal, (2) essentially normal, (3) abnormal, or (4) technically insufficient. The last is reserved for when artifact or other technical limitations prevent answering the clinical question at hand. "Essentially normal" is reserved for situations when findings have two or more alternative explanations that result from either normal or abnormal processes. Slowing of the frequency of alpha rhythm, for example, can result from either drowsiness or mild encephalopathy, and insufficient documentation may make these choices ambiguous.

In the current case, the patient spent the first half of the recording with restless wakefulness, and the second with intermittent drowsiness, when EEG activities were less obscured by artifact. As opposed to diffuse enhanced beta activity from medication effects, muscle artifact is localized to involved muscles. Whereas abnormally enhanced beta activities are present throughout the recording, muscle artifact varies with state and patient activities.

Clinical Pearls

1. Variable beta activities >25 cps likely result from EMG activity and can obscure interpretation of the tracing.

2. Technologists may improve artifact by patient manipulation. Sleep or sedation may be required in uncooperative subjects.

3. EEG reports must state that the recording is normal, abnormal, essentially normal, or technically insufficient.

PATIENT 12

A 51-year-old woman with spells of diaphoresis and unresponsiveness

A 51-year-old woman is evaluated for risk of epileptic seizures after she had several spells of diaphoresis, tachypnea, and subsequent unresponsiveness. She is taking no medications.

The patient was instructed to stay up all night before the recording. The EEG was recorded with the patient awake.

Question: What are the posterior sharp transients called that occur after eye opening *(arrows at enlarged inset)?*

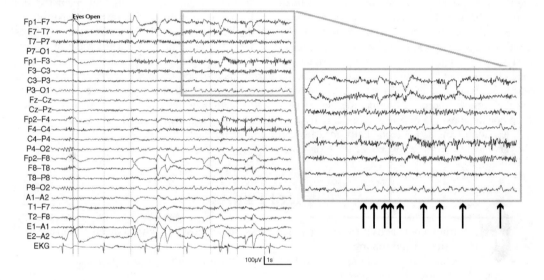

Answer: Sporadic positive waves present in occipital channels during eye opening are called *lambda waves* and are findings designating saccades.

Discussion: In contrast to eye movements that generate artifact, *lambda waves* are cerebral activities that correspond to the saccades that accompany visual fixation and scanning.

They usually appear as irregular trains of biphasic, sharp, surface-positive potentials in occipital channels. Although, in the example, they do not exceed 30 μV, they can be quite prominent in children. Lambda waves can also be polyphasic with a prominent negative deflection. The appearance of lambda waves decreases with increasing age.

Brightly illuminated rooms can exacerbate their appearance. The technologist can differentiate them from pathologic sharp waves by demonstrating their dependence on bright room lighting or their appearance with visual scanning.

In this particular case, the recording was performed following partial *sleep deprivation.*

Sleep deprivation serves three purposes. First, sleep deprivation is an accepted *activation procedure.* Activation procedures attempt to increase the yield of IEDs in susceptible individuals. Most studies have shown that yield of IEDs increases following sleep deprivation.

Second, sleep deprivation promotes the occurrence of sleep. Sleep itself is an important activation procedure, because certain epilepsy syndromes have IEDs that appear more frequently during certain sleep-wake states. Sleep and sleep deprivation have cumulative effects in increasing the yield of IEDs.

Sleep also improves the quality of recordings in lieu of sedation. Chloral hydrate was the standard agent for sedation of uncooperative patients during EEG, largely for the belief that it had little effect on normal activities or on the incidence of IEDs. Studies show no clear morbidity related to use of chloral hydrate for pediatric sedation in EEG, but cases of mortality or morbidity have been reported for overdoses. Some laboratories encourage use of mild sedatives, such as melatonin or diphenhydramine, instead of chloral hydrate. Such "conscious sedation" requires the training of staff in resuscitation and monitoring of vital signs, or scheduling physician-supervised anesthesia during procedures.

Heightened concerns over medical liability and increasing requirements for specialized training and monitoring make routine sedation impractical for most laboratories. This shift in practice appears for the better, with some authorities reporting no clear changes in the rates in unsuccessful tests, despite a drastic drop in sedation use. Sleep deprivation, sleep, and judicious scheduling of potentially uncooperative patients in the afternoon (when circadian cycles and sleep deprivation make it a time of day especially favorable to sleep) have supplanted pharmacologic sedation in many U.S. laboratories.

Clinical Pearls

1. Lambda waves are sharp, transient, surface positive discharges accompanying saccadic eye movement during visual scanning.

2. As we will see in subsequent cases, "sharpness" is not synonymous with epilepsy. Benign findings can have a sharp morphology.

3. Sleep and sleep deprivation can activate the appearance of IEDs.

4. Sleep and sleep deprivation are important replacements for sedation once routinely used for recording EEGs in children and uncooperative patients.

REFERENCES

1. Cote CJ, Karl HW, Notterman DA, et al: Adverse sedation events in pediatrics: Analysis of medications used for sedation. Pediatrics 2000; 106:633–644.
2. Fountain NB, Kim JS, Lee SI: Sleep deprivation activates epileptiform discharges independent of the activating effects of sleep. J Clin Neurophysiol 1998; 15(1):69–75.
3. Olson DM, Sheehan MG, Thompson W, et al: Sedation of children for electroencephalograms. Pediatrics 2001; 108:163–165.
4. Roth M, Green J: The lambda wave as a normal physiological phenomenon in the human electroencephalogram. Nature 1953; 172:864–866.
5. Thoresen M, Henriksen O, Wannag E, et al: Does a sedative dose of chloral hydrate modify the EEG of children with epilepsy?. Electroencephalogr Clin Neurophysiol 1997; 102:152–157.

PATIENT 13

A 4-year-old girl with headaches and inattention

A 4-year-old girl has been sent home on numerous occasions for diffuse headaches and inattention. The referring physician is considering absence seizures.

The child is awake, hyperventilating, and taking no medications. The child initially refuses hyperventilation but successfully performs when asked to blow on a pinwheel. Eye leads are omitted because of poor cooperation.

Question: What is the finding in the following tracing?

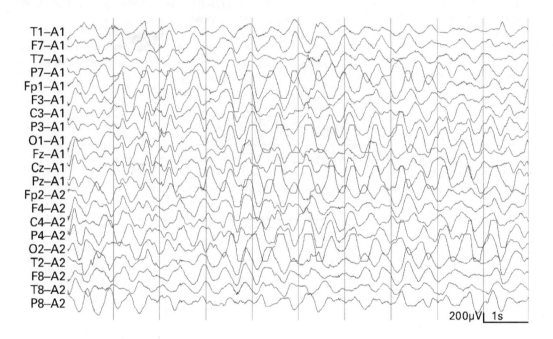

Answer: The recording shows a burst of diffusely distributed, rhythmic, high-amplitude 2 cps delta activity induced by hyperventilation. This response is normal "buildup."

Discussion: Hyperventilation for one or two 3- to 4-minute trials is a routine activation procedure. The term *buildup* is the term for the slowing that emerges from central nervous system (CNS) blood flow changes induced by hypocapnia. In children, buildup often takes the form of high-amplitude, generalized, synchronous, symmetric rhythmic delta activity. Less impressive responses, such as emergence of low-amplitude bursts of symmetric theta activity, can be present in older children or adults. Adults often have no discernible changes.

Seizures in susceptible patients are the only unequivocal abnormalities induced by hyperventilation.

Other findings during hyperventilation must be interpreted in context.

Asymmetric or focal slowing limited to hyperventilation is a relative abnormality that indicates subtle dysfunction over the side with more severe slowing.

Persistent buildup, that which lasts over a minute following cessation of hyperventilation, is thought by some to be a nonspecific abnormality, but persistent slowing or marked buildup can result from hypoglycemia. The EEG technologist should note routinely the time of the patient's last meal, and, if buildup is remarkable in duration, a retrial is often performed after administration of a glucose-containing snack.

Hyperventilation is avoided in those with cardiovascular or neurovascular disease because vasoconstriction is a possible result of hypocapnia.

Clinical Pearls

1. Hyperventilation is a routine activation procedure that is most useful in provoking absence seizures.
2. Buildup is the symmetric slowing induced by hyperventilation-induced hypocapnia.

PATIENT 14

A 14-year-old girl with spells of headaches and confusion

A 14-year-old girl has headaches and confusion thought to be consistent with atypical migraine or complex partial seizures.

The recording was performed with the patient awake and on no medications. This portion is recorded during intermittent photic stimulation, with each flash of a strobe light indicated by the tic marks in the photic channel.

Question: What does the response in the tracing shown below, during photic stimulation, indicate?

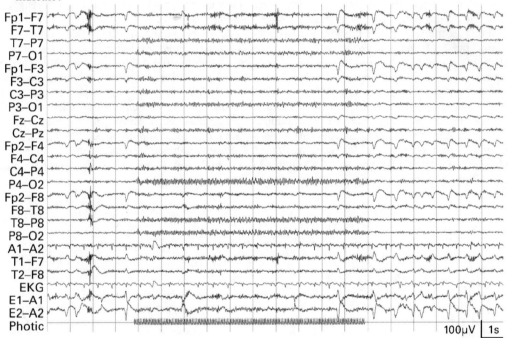

Answer: The burst of occipital activity following the frequency of the photic stimulation is a normal driving response to photic driving.

Discussion: Intermittent photic stimulation is a standard activation procedure. Although various protocols are used, usually patients are exposed to a series of 10-second blocks of stimulation at frequencies starting at 2 Hz and increasing to 20 Hz, before decreasing again to 2 Hz. Many centers repeat stimulation with eyes open and closed. Others expose patients to blocks of gradually and continuously increasing or decreasing flash frequencies.

The normal response to photic stimulation is a *symmetric driving response*, a rhythmic occipital or posteriorly dominant activity that occurs at the primary frequency or at a slower harmonic to the rate of the flashes. Sometimes a brief burst of sharp activity with onset or offset of stimulation occurs, a normal "on-response" or "off-response." Subharmonic driving and an on-response are shown on the second example taken from another patient. Driving responses need not be continuous throughout the stimulation. Indeed, the "on-response" in this example (as well as other published examples) may consist of a fragment of rhythmic photic driving.

Another normal response is the lack of photic driving.

Photomyoclonus (photomyogenic) responses are the twitching of facial and sometimes upper trunk muscles in response to each flash. No epileptic discharges accompany photomyoclonus, but anterior muscle artifacts may be present. It is best thought of as an exaggerated startle response. Some observe that photomyoclonus may appear during the acute phase of alcohol withdrawal and may be evidence of sympathetic hyperactivity.

The only unequivocally abnormal response to intermittent photic stimulation is a triggered epileptic seizure.

A more common abnormal finding is a *photoparoxysmal response*, a burst of asymptomatic generalized multiple spike-wave discharges.

Other relative abnormalities include asymmetry, during which driving responses are present on one side and absent on the other. Its significance, however, is limited in the absence of corroborating focal abnormalities.

High-amplitude responses or high-amplitude occipital spikes are seen in neuronal ceroid lipofuscinosis.

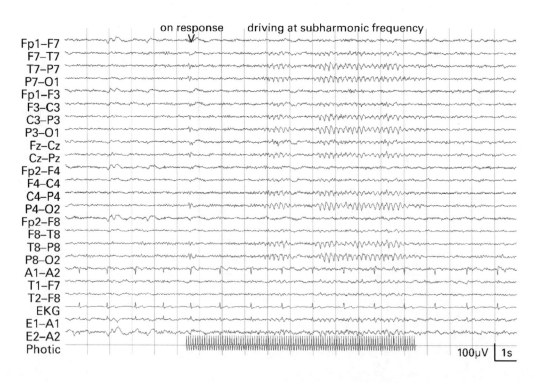

Clinical Pearls

1. Intermittent photic stimulation is an activation procedure intended to induce interictal epileptiform discharges or seizures in susceptible individuals.

2. Normal results of intermittent photic stimulation include symmetric photic driving or lack of responses.

3. Photomyoclonus is an exaggerated, nonepileptic motor response to photic stimulation.

4. Photoparoxysmal responses consist of generalized polyspike-wave discharges in response to photic driving.

REFERENCE

1. Trenite DG, Binnie CD, Harding GF, et al: Medical technology assessment photic stimulation—Standardization of screening methods. Neurophysiol Clin 1999; 29:318–324.

PATIENT 15

A 23-year-old woman undergoing overnight video-EEG recordings (Part 1)

A 23-year-old woman undergoes overnight video-EEG recordings for diagnosis of spells of unknown etiology. A baseline recording while awake is normal, featuring a 10-cps alpha rhythm. The patient is taking no medications.

Questions: What is the source of the phase-reversing slow waves seen best at F7 and F8 *(arrows)*? In what state is this patient?

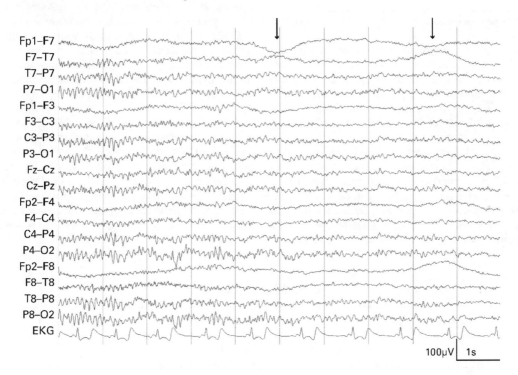

Answers: The source of the slow waves is lateral eye movements. The patient is in a state of drowsiness (stage 1 sleep).

Discussion: Polysomnography (PSG) is required for formal sleep scoring. PSG, with the use of central and occipital EEG electrodes, eye movement leads, and EMG leads, assigns one of six sleep stages to 30-second epochs of data. These stages are as follows:

Common		Predominant		
Stage	Name	EEG Frequency	Eye Movement	EMG
Stage W	Wakeful-ness	Alpha	++	++
1	Drowsi-ness	Theta	slow rolling	+
2	Light sleep	Theta	−	+
3 and 4	Deep sleep	Delta	−	+
REM	REM sleep	Alpha/theta	++	−

REM, rapid eye movement.

Stages 1–4 are often grouped together as non-REM sleep. During a normal duration of nocturnal sleep, most healthy adults spend about 75% of time in non-REM sleep and 25% in REM sleep. Sleep stages typically occur in brief episodes tied to a 90- to 110-minute ultradian (less than 1 day) cycle.

Although formal sleep scoring is inappropriate to undertake on the data usually acquired with clinical EEG, it is important to recognize characteristic changes of state so that they can be distinguished from pathologic changes. In fact, to interpret EEG, the interpreter must know unambiguously what clinical state the patient is in during the recording.

Several features identify the adult drowsy state in the previous tracing.

Slowing or attenuation of the alpha rhythm from the patient's normal waking posterior rhythm denotes drowsiness. In some patients, the frequency gradually slows; in others, it abruptly attenuates and is replaced by theta activity.

Emergence of diffusely distributed theta activities. In formal sleep scoring, more than 50% of a 30-second epoch must consist of theta activity.

Slow lateral eye movements, seen as ~0.5 cps slow waves in the anterior channels of this example, commonly occur with the transition to and the onset of sleep.

Note that no eye leads were used on this study. Because most patients remain on intensive monitoring for several days instead of the standard 8 hours of routine PSG, eye leads are used only if there are particular questions to answer. Even then, facial skin is sensitive, and eye leads are only placed short term. Lateral eye movements usually cause phase reversals best seen in electrodes F7 or F8, helpful evidence when eye leads are absent.

Other findings common in drowsiness include transient enhancement of beta activity. Hypersynchrony (brief bursts of generalized delta activity during light sleep) are often present in children and young adults. Benign interictal epileptiform discharges—sharp waves without pathologic correlates—often appear during drowsiness or light sleep. Bursts of theta activities, usually generalized but sometimes with a left or right hemispheric prominence, occur from time to time.

Drowsiness is distinguished from mild encephalopathy by its transient nature; the EEG technologist should stimulate the patient to demonstrate arousal (and normal waking activities) to provide a comparison.

Clinical Pearls

1. Drowsiness (stage 1 sleep) is marked by attenuation or slowing of alpha rhythm, emergence of diffusely distributed theta activities, and, in some cases, slow rolling, lateral eye movements and enhancement of beta activities.

2. Arousal and return to normal waking activities distinguishes normal drowsiness from mild encephalopathy.

REFERENCE

1. Rechtschaffen A, Kales A: A Manual of Standardized Terminology, Techniques, and Scoring System for Sleep Stages of Human Subjects. Los Angeles, Brain Information Service, Brain Research Institute, UCLA, 1968.

PATIENT 16

A 23-year-old woman undergoing overnight video-EEG recordings (Part 2)

This excerpt from the same patient is taken 5 minutes after the previous sample.

Questions: Name the diffusely distributed findings at times *a* and *b* and the occipital transients at *c*. In what state is the patient?

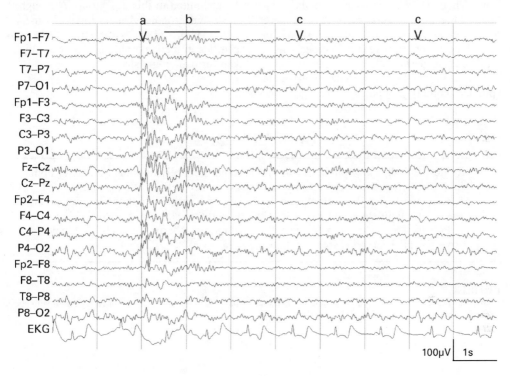

Answers: (a) K complex; (b) sleep spindle; (c) positive occipital sharp transients of sleep. The patient is in light sleep (stage 2 sleep).

Discussion: The predominant frequency during stage 2 sleep (light sleep) is theta activity, although delta activities may appear intermittently.

Stage 2 sleep is defined as the first appearance of sleep spindles. *Sleep spindles* are symmetric, synchronous bursts of 11–14 cps activities, with maximal amplitudes in central regions. Durations in adults typically remain between 1 and 3 seconds. Sleep spindles have characteristic spindle-form morphology with amplitudes at the beginning and end of each burst being smaller than the midportion. Although their appearance defines stage 2 sleep, they often appear in deeper stages of non-REM sleep but are harder to see because of state-related changes in background activity.

K complexes are high-amplitude, biphasic or polyphasic centrally dominant discharges that emerge during stage 2 sleep. Sleep spindles can appear at the end of a K complex, as seen in this case. Vertex sharp transients, another characteristic midline finding during sleep, can also appear near or linked to K complexes. K complexes are frequently evoked by auditory stimulation, such as noise in the hallway outside of the EEG recording room.

Positive occipital sharp transients of sleep (POSTS) may occur during stage 1 or 2 sleep. They appear most commonly in young adults but are not limited to this age group. Although they appear synchronously in occipital channels, the amplitudes are often asymmetric. Their importance lies in their morphology; they can be mistaken for pathologic sharp waves.

Clinical Pearls

1. Sleep spindles are spindle-form, synchronous, centrally dominant bursts of high alpha- or low-frequency beta activity. Their appearance defines stage 2 sleep.

2. K complexes are high amplitude, biphasic or polyphasic midline discharges that appear during light sleep and can be evoked by auditory stimuli.

3. POSTS are bisynchronous, usually asymmetric, sharp transients that have a positive potential recorded from occipital regions.

REFERENCE
1. Loomis AL, Harvey EN, Hobart G: Distribution of disturbance patterns in the human electroencephalogram with special reference to sleep. J Neurophysiol 1938; 1:413–430.

PATIENT 17

A 23-year-old woman undergoing overnight video-EEG recordings (Part 3)

This excerpt, taken from the same monitoring session as the previous two samples, is recorded 15 minutes after the first excerpt.

Question: In what state is this patient?

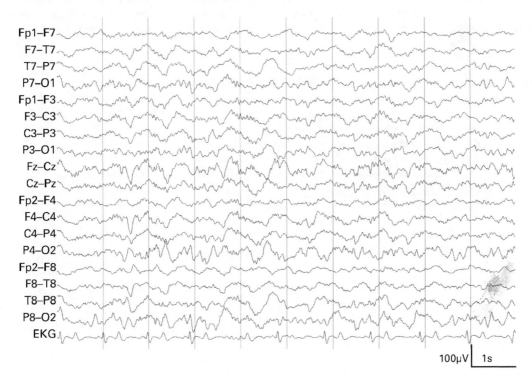

Answer: Deep sleep (stages 3–4 sleep).

Discussion: The predominance of delta activities defines sleep stages 3 and 4 (*deep sleep, slow wave sleep*). Delta activities in stages 3–4 sleep appear as semirhythmic, generalized delta activities with amplitudes = 75 μV. Sleep spindles, K complexes, vertex sharp transients, and other mixed frequencies can also be present but may be less easily distinguishable from high-amplitude delta activities.

Formal sleep scoring with the use of PSG restricts delta activity to those activities = 2 cps that = 75 μV in amplitude obtained in specific central and occipital channels referred to contra-lateral references (C3-A2, O1-A2, C4-A1, O2-A1). Stage 3 is defined when delta activity occupies 20–50% of a 30-second epoch and stage 4 more than 50% of an epoch.

Because most clinical EEG is performed during the day, and because sleep usually starts with stage 1 sleep, deep sleep is rarely seen in the daytime realm of the typical EEG lab. Slow wave sleep is commonplace, however, during overnight recordings in epilepsy monitoring units. The recognition of deep sleep is important because delta activities may be present in cases of moderate to severe encephalopathy.

Clinical Pearls

1. Stages 3 and 4 are defined as the appearance of = 75 μV, semirhythmic generalized delta activities during sleep.

2. Sleep scoring uses a more restrictive definition of the delta frequency band (≤2 cps = 75 μV) than clinical EEG (<4 cps, no amplitude criteria).

3. Delta activity in stage 3 sleep must occupy 20–50% of the epoch, whereas stage 4 sleep >50%.

PATIENT 18

A 23-year-old woman undergoing overnight video-EEG recordings (Part 4)

This excerpt from the same patient is taken another 20 minutes after the previous sample. The patient is taking no medications.

Questions: Name the findings marked at the arrows. In what state is this patient?

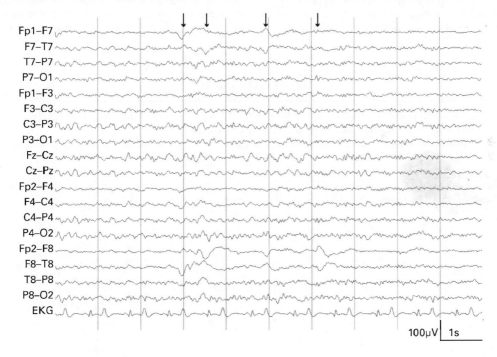

Answers: The finding marked at the arrows is REMs. The patient is in REM sleep.

Discussion: REM sleep is formally defined as a state during which rapid eye movements appear during EEG activities of low amplitude, asynchronous, generalized mixed alpha and theta activities, and during hypotonia measured by submental EMG. REMs are quick, saccade-like movements, unlike the slow lateral movements seen in drowsiness. They typically appear in bursts and, conversely, may be absent for long stretches of REM sleep, requiring the formulation of so-called "REM rules" in sleep scoring to increase consistency.

REM hypotonia, determined by the lack of muscle activity in submental EMG leads, is present and important in distinction of REM from light sleep or wakefulness.

REM sleep is sometimes called *paradoxical sleep* because the desynchronized, low-amplitude, mixed alpha and theta activities appear more similar to those of wakefulness than the slower, more synchronized activities of non-REM sleep.

Like slow-wave sleep, REM sleep is seldom encountered in standard clinical EEG laboratory. The mean latency of onset of REM exceeds 20 minutes in healthy adults. Sleep onset REM, however, can be seen after severe sleep deprivation or in primary sleep disorders, such as narcolepsy.

Clinical Pearl

REM sleep is defined by the appearance of REMs, hypotonia, and desynchronized, low-amplitude, mixed theta, and alpha frequency activities.

REFERENCE

1. Rechtschaffen A, Kales A: A Manual of Standardized Terminology, Techniques, and Scoring System for Sleep Stages of Human Subjects. Los Angeles, Brain Information Service, Brain Research Institute, UCLA, 1968.

PATIENT 19

A 30-year-old woman with depression with psychotic features

An EEG is requested to evaluate possible encephalopathy in a 30-year-old woman with major depression with psychotic features, who was scheduled for electroconvulsive therapy (ECT). Medications were haloperidol and mirtazapine.

The recording is made with the patient asleep.

Questions: Do diffuse beta activities on the early portion of the sample *(under bar)* indicate medication effects? What is the transient present at Cz at the arrow?

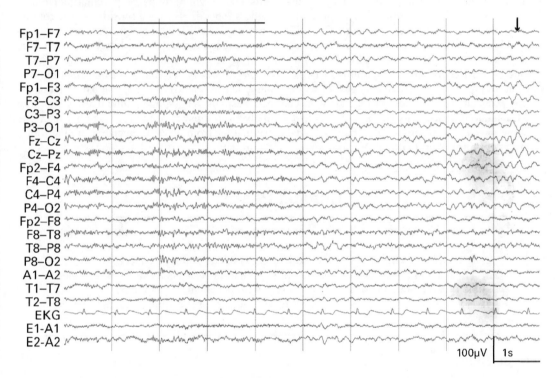

Answers: Beta activities of drowsiness are normal. Present at Cz is a vertex sharp transient of sleep.

Discussion: Beta activities may become transiently enhanced during drowsiness or light sleep. They should be symmetric and diffusely distributed. Enhanced beta activities, because of drug ingestion, on the other hand, should be present throughout the tracing regardless of state.

The EEG is sensitive in detection of encephalopathies—states of altered consciousness or delirium. Psychiatric diseases largely spare the level of consciousness. Thus, the main use of EEG in the evaluation of psychiatric diseases is to evaluate possible encephalopathy that may be difficult to distinguish from primary psychiatric disease. In the case of treatment of depression with ECT, EEG may aid in screening of organic causes of depression that may not respond to ECT. Following ECT, EEG may aid in determining whether clinical responses stem from changes in mood versus postictal confusion or complications, such as ECT-induced nonconvulsive status epilepticus.

Some psychiatric disorders may be associated with epileptiform abnormalities. Various studies find that benign epileptiform variants are often seen in patients with schizophrenia or depression. Other studies have attempted to use digital EEG techniques to map out the distributions of the various frequency bands that may be characteristic of certain psychiatric diseases. Critics of these studies point out that statistical techniques, data and subject selection, and other experimental problems make these studies controversial. It is clear, however, that the broad overlap of EEG findings between psychiatric patients and controls and within groups of psychiatric patients renders specificity and sensitivity of routine EEG or digital EEG techniques too low for diagnostic use in the evaluation of specific psychiatric diseases.

The current patient has a normal EEG, indicating to her psychiatrists that her apparent lethargy, poor responsiveness, and hallucinations are more likely from a psychiatric process rather than one originating from an unappreciated organic brain syndrome.

Clinical Pearls

1. Beta activities may be briefly enhanced in amplitude during drowsiness or light sleep.

2. Beta activities must be interpreted in context of the patient's state.

3. The main use of EEG in evaluation of psychiatric disease is its ability to evaluate possible organic brain syndromes that present with psychiatric symptoms.

4. No commonly accepted, specific EEG findings are attributed to psychiatric disease.

REFERENCES

1. Hughes J: A review of the usefulness of the standard EEG in psychiatry. Clin Electroencephalogr 1996; 27(1): 35–39.
2. Inui K, Motomura E, Okushima R, et al: Electroencephalographic findings in patients with DSM-IV mood disorder, schizophrenia, other psychotic disorders. Biol Psychiatry 1998; 43(1): 69–75.
3. John ER, Prichep LS, Fridman J, Easton P: Neurometrics: Computer-assisted differential diagnosis of brain dysfunctions. Science 1998; 239(4836): 162–169.
4. Oken B, Chiappa K: Statistical issues concerning computerized analysis of brainwave topography. Ann Neurol 1986; 19: 493–494.

PATIENT 20

A 22-year-old man with intermittent confusion

A 22-year-old man presents with intermittent confusion. The patient takes olanzapine.

The EEG is performed after the patient has improved clinically. He is asleep for most of the recording.

Question: What are the sources and clinical significance of sharp transients at points *a, b,* and *c*?

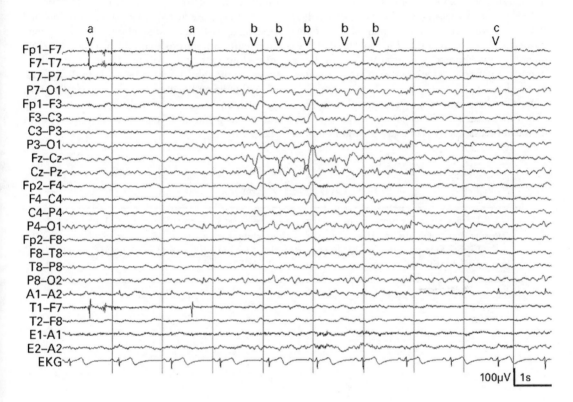

Answer: (a) electrode pop at F7, (b) vertex sharp transients of sleep, (c) POSTS. None of these findings is abnormal.

Discussion: Distinctions among IEDs, sharp artifacts, and normal sharp transients are some of the main challenges of EEG interpretation.

Electrode pop. Electrode pops are transient capacitive discharges caused by abnormalities of the electrode-scalp interface. Pops are easily identified because of their short duration (<20 milliseconds), extremely sharp biphasic morphology, confinement to a single electrode, and the characteristic that, rather than interrupting ongoing activity, they appear upon it.

Vertex sharp transients of sleep. Also called "vertex sharp waves," they, along with K complexes and sleep spindles, form a triad of frequently encountered, centrally or midline dominant patterns associated with lighter stages of sleep.

Vertex sharp waves are large-amplitude (75–150 µV) transients. Vertex sharp waves in children can be especially remarkable, attaining high amplitudes and occurring in brief, semirhythmic trains. They are located at the central vertex with a symmetric, diffusely distributed field. Some patients may show shifting of maximum potential from side to side, but consistently asymmetrically distributed vertex sharp waves indicate subtle hemispheric dysfunction of the underrepresented hemisphere. Note that inaccurate electrode placement can also lead to this finding.

The morphology of vertex sharp waves helps in their distinction from midline IEDs. Vertex sharp waves are usually broad in duration and V-shaped, with an initial abrupt negativity and an equally abrupt positive return to baseline. No after-slow potentials occur after vertex sharp waves, although care must be made to distinguish normal theta and delta activities of sleep that may by happenstance occur behind a vertex sharp wave. Sleep spindles frequently occur after vertex sharp waves.

Clinical Pearls

1. Vertex sharp waves are high-amplitude, symmetric, vertex-dominant sharp discharges that occur during drowsiness and light sleep.

2. Light sleep presents multiple opportunities for sharp transients of sleep and other benign epileptiform discharges to be confused with IEDs.

PATIENT 21

A 7-month-old infant with concern of seizures

An EEG is requested because of a concern of seizures in a 7-month-old male infant with shaking spells several times a week and one staring spell 3 weeks prior. The patient takes no medications.

Questions: In what stage sleep is this child? Are the findings indicative of this stage normal for age?

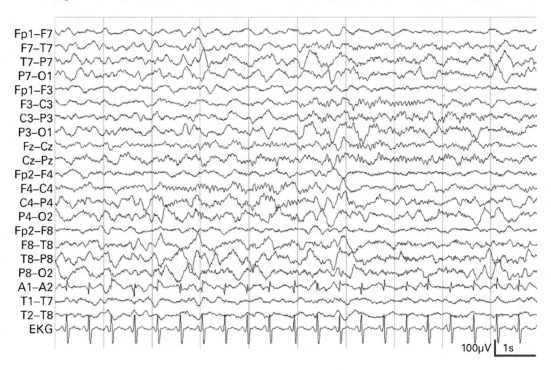

Answers: Stage 2 sleep, identified by sleep spindles. Prolonged, asynchronous sleep spindles are normal for this age.

Discussion: The characteristics of sleep spindles change with age.

Sleep spindles begin to appear during continuous, non-REM sleep at ages 2–3 months, about the same time of onset of the posteriorly dominant waking rhythm. The duration of sleep spindles in infants is usually around 3–4 seconds, but they can be also markedly prolonged, as seen in this case, attaining durations of about 10 seconds. Sleep spindles of adults, on the other hand, seldom exceed 3–4 seconds.

Sleep spindles in infants and toddlers appear asynchronously. Although asynchronous, the overall persistence from side to side should equal out over the course of the tracing. Although early sleep spindles are asynchronous, they should always be symmetric in amplitude.

Sleep spindles usually become synchronous by age 1. Asynchronous sleep spindles beyond age 2 are abnormal, possibly indicating defects in interhemispheric connections, such as abnormal development of the corpus callosum.

Clinical Pearls

1. Sleep spindles first appear at ages 2–3 months, in parallel with onset of the posteriorly dominant waking rhythm.

2. Sleep spindles can be asynchronous until age 2 but should always be symmetric in amplitude and in overall persistence from side to side.

PATIENT 22

A 7-year-old boy with inattentive spells

A 7-year-old boy has spells of inattention unresponsive to stimulant therapy for attention-deficit disorder. The patient takes Dexedrine.

The patient is asleep throughout most of the study.

Question: Identify the following finding recorded in the transition from drowsiness to light sleep.

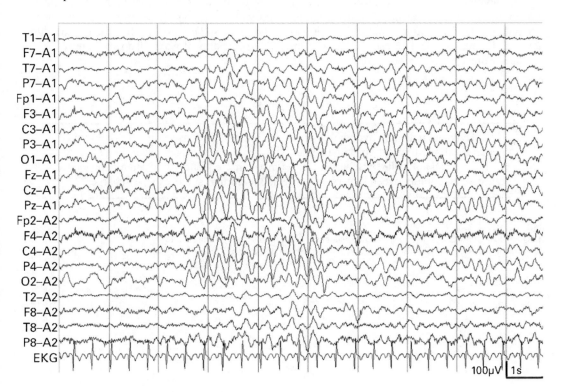

Answer: The recording shows a burst of generalized, rhythmic 4 cps delta activities, a normal finding of infancy and childhood during the transition from wakefulness to sleep, or hypnagogic hypersynchrony.

Discussion: Hypersynchrony of drowsiness occurs either during transition from wakefulness to sleep (hypnagogic hypersynchrony) or from sleep to wakefulness (hypnopompic hypersynchrony). Hypersynchrony consists of bursts of generalized, rhythmic, 4 cps delta activities. Hypersynchrony first emerges about the time a waking posterior rhythm first develops at age 3 months. The peak age of expression is between ages 6 months and 1 year. Nevertheless, hypersynchrony is often present in older children through age 12. Its incidence fades through adolescence but may be rarely present up to the third decade of life.

Hypersynchrony may be misidentified as abnormal epileptic discharges. Faster frequencies of ongoing background activity are often superimposed on the burst of delta activities, giving the false appearance of spike-wave discharges. Unlike spike-wave discharges, however, the apparent "spikes" have no clear relationship to the phase of the slow-wave components. The frequency of hypersynchrony, usually about 4 cps, is unusual for spike-wave bursts in epilepsy. Furthermore, hypersynchrony, in contrast to abnormal spike-wave discharges, is seen during these transitional wake-sleep states only.

Pearls

1. Hypnagogic and hypnopompic hypersynchrony consist of high-amplitude, generalized, rhythmic, 4-cps bursts of activity seen in transitional wake-drowsy states.
2. The lack of spike discharges, differences in frequency, and state-dependence allow distinction between hypersynchrony and abnormal spike-wave discharges.

REFERENCES
1. Gibbs FA, Gibbs EL: Atlas of Electroencephalography. Cambridge, MA, Addison-Wesley, 1952.
2. Santamaria J, Chiappa KE: The EEG of Drowsiness. New York, Demos Publications, 1987.

The EEG undergoes characteristic changes that echo the rapid development of the neonatal brain. To document these changes and determine their appropriate occurrence, neonatal recordings have specific technical requirements. Acquisition differs in three respects.

First, neonatal recordings require polygraphic data. These data are EEG, eye movement electrodes, respiration thermosisters or thoracic strain gauges, EMG, and EKG. Polygraphic data are required to match the determination of activity state and developmentally appropriate background EEG activity.

Second, the small size of the neonatal head may prevent the use of the full 10–20 electrode coverage. Fp3-4 electrodes (halfway between Fp and F) are commonly used, and frontal and parietal electrodes may be omitted. This results in electrodes that are 40% rather than 20% of the primary head measurements.

Third, neonatal recordings are performed for a minimum of 1 hour rather than the 20 minutes for older subjects. The cycling of sleep-wake states in the neonate is much faster (50–60 minutes) than that of older children and adults (24 hours). The extended recording time allows the occurrence of at least one spontaneous change in state.

Unlike adult sleep scoring, epoch duration or paper speed in neonatal polygraphy is not rigidly defined. To facilitate interpretation of polygraphic data, many acquire neonatal recordings at one-half to one-third paper speed (15–10 mm/s) and use epoch durations of 30 seconds to 1 minute. Digital systems are obviously suited for neonatal studies, given the ability to change paper speed (page width) as needed.

Interpretation of a neonatal recording requires calculation of the estimated conceptional age (ECA):

$$ECA = \text{estimated gestational age} + \text{postpartum age}.$$

The healthy neonate meets a timetable of developmental changes matched to ECA. The term *neonate* has three basic activity states: wakefulness, active sleep, and quiet sleep.

Activity		Background			
State	Observation	EEG Pattern	EOG	EMG	Respiration
Wakefulness	Body movements Eyes open	Continuous	++	Phasic Tonic	Irregular
Active sleep	Irregular body movements Eyes closed	Continuous	++	Phasic Hypotonic	Irregular
Quiet sleep	No movement Eyes open	Discontinuous and continuous	–	Tonic	Regular

Wakefulness is defined by the observation of open eyes, agitation, or crying. Technologist's notes and eye leads that demonstrate spontaneous eye opening are the most reliable polygraphic findings in wakefulness. *Quiet sleep* is the immature precursor to non-REM sleep. Quiet sleep is distinguished on polygraphic channels as periods of little muscle activity, no eye movements, and rhythmic breathing. *Active sleep* is the precursor to REM sleep and, as in REM sleep, is defined by rapid eye movements. Other findings on polygraphic channels are irregular respirations, eye movements, and decreased EMG tone.

At an early stage of development, premature neonates can spend more than 50% of time in active sleep. As infants mature, the persistence of active sleep decreases. Unlike adult sleep, which starts with non-REM sleep, active sleep initiates sleep in neonates. Active sleep may be difficult to distinguish from wakefulness because of similarities of EEG findings.

A practical goal of any neonatal recording is to document the occurrence of at least one change in activity state. State change is an essential finding in neonatal recording, because its absence is an important indicator of encephalopathy.

The background EEG activities of a neonate that accompany activity states (and change with maturation) are of two basic types: discontinuous and continuous.

Discontinuous activities consist of low-amplitude activities that are recurrently interrupted by periodic bursts of higher-amplitude activities. If >50% of a 1-minute epoch consists of higher-amplitude activities, some designate the background as *semidiscontinuous*. The duration between bursts decreases with ECA. Discontinuous activities are seen in premature infants (*tracé discontinu* [TD]) and persist as a part of quiet sleep in more mature infants (*tracé alternant* [TA]).

Continuous activities are mixed-frequency activities that do not feature the abrupt changes of amplitude of discontinuous activities. Continuous activities emerge reliably at ECA 30 weeks and become the main background activities of wakefulness and active sleep. Continuous activities of wakefulness and active sleep are often classified further, but the nomenclature is inconsistent. *Activité moyenne, mixed activities, low voltage irregular* (LVI), and *tracé continu* all refer to low-amplitude, rather featureless, mixed activities with varying predominance of delta, theta, and alpha frequency activities. In this text, those described previously will be referred to simply as *continuous activities*.

A final subtype of continuous activities consists of semirhythmic, medium- to high-amplitude delta activities termed *high voltage slow* (HVS) or *tracé continu lentement)*, which are seen in quiet sleep of full-term neonates.

Various *physiologic EEG patterns* appear at different steps of maturation, help in confirming ECA, and aid in differentiating background activities. In Figure 6-1, the first appearance, maximal expression, and resolution of specific patterns are represented by the gray polygons within each vertical column.

Discordance between ECA and expected EEG findings that exceeds 2 weeks is a finding termed *dysmaturity*. Dysmaturity indicates encephalopathy or serves as a warning that the ECA was misstated. Figure 6-1 details various developmental stages, which are reviewed in subsequent cases.

Question: Why are background EEG activities often designated in French?

Answer: French investigators, headed by C. Dreyfus-Brisac and colleagues (see following reference for an excellent review), have a long and respected history of the description of the normal neonatal EEG and its deviation in pathologic states. Accordingly, this history persists in the use of *les môts justes* in its description.

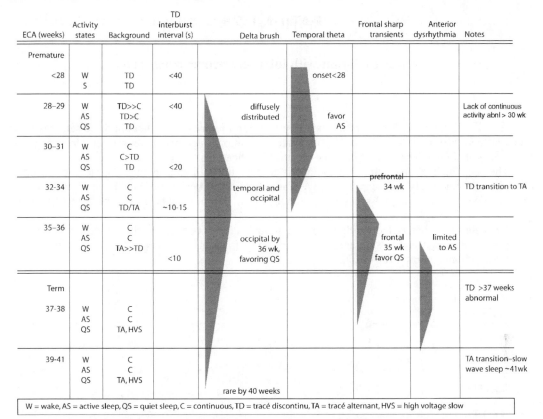

ECA (weeks)	Activity states	Background	TD interburst interval (s)	Delta brush	Temporal theta	Frontal sharp transients	Anterior dysrhythmia	Notes
Premature <28	W S	TD TD	<40		onset<28			
28–29	W AS QS	TD>>C TD>C TD	<40	diffusely distributed	favor AS			Lack of continuous activity abnl > 30 wk
30–31	W AS QS	C C>TD TD	<20					
32-34	W AS QS	C C TD/TA	~10-15	temporal and occipital		prefrontal 34 wk		TD transition to TA
35–36	W AS QS	C C TA>>TD	<10	occipital by 36 wk, favoring QS		frontal 35 wk favor QS	limited to AS	
Term 37-38	W AS QS	C C TA, HVS						TD >37 weeks abnormal
39-41	W AS QS	C C TA, HVS		rare by 40 weeks				TA transition–slow wave sleep ~41wk

W = wake, AS = active sleep, QS = quiet sleep, C = continuous, TD = tracé discontinu, TA = tracé alternant, HVS = high voltage slow

Figure 6-1. The first appearance, maximal expression, and resolution of specific patterns are represented by the gray polygons within each vertical column.

Clinical Pearls

1. Neonatal polygraphy uses a subset of scalp electrodes, EMG, respiratory, cardiac, and eye movement monitoring and is performed for at least 1 hour.

2. ECA = estimated gestational age + postpartum age. Findings in neonatal EEG are keyed to ECA.

3. The three basic activity states of neonates are wakefulness, active sleep, and quiet sleep.

4. Background EEG activities of neonates are classified as discontinuous or continuous.

5. A lag of expected EEG changes for a given ECA is termed *dysmaturity* and is one sign of encephalopathy.

REFERENCES

1. Guideline 2: Minimum technical requirements for performing pediatric electroencephalography. J Clin Neurophysiol 1994; 3:7–11.
2. Lamblin MD, d'Allest AM, André M, et al: EEG in premature and full-term infants: Developmental features and glossary. Neurophysiol Clin 1999; 29:1232–1219.
3. Werner SS, Stockard JE, Bickford RG: Atlas of Neonatal Electroencephalography. New York, Raven Press, 1977.

PATIENT 23

Premature infant with intraventricular hemorrhage

An EEG is requested to determine possible ongoing motor activity thought to be seizures in an infant at day 25 postpartum who has an estimated gestational age of 23 weeks. An intraventricular hemorrhage is found. The patient is on no sedative medications.

The technologist notes that the patient is asleep and still during this sample. The child is breathing spontaneously on a ventilator. Eye leads are omitted because of nursing staff request. The same sample is shown with a 3-second page (paper speed 10 mm/s) and a 10-second page (30 mm/s).

Questions: What is the estimated conceptional age? Name the background activity of this premature infant and the findings at the arrows (shown at a reduced sensitivity in inset). Are these findings normal for this age?

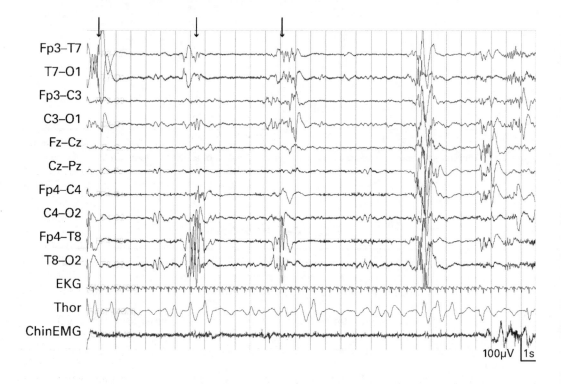

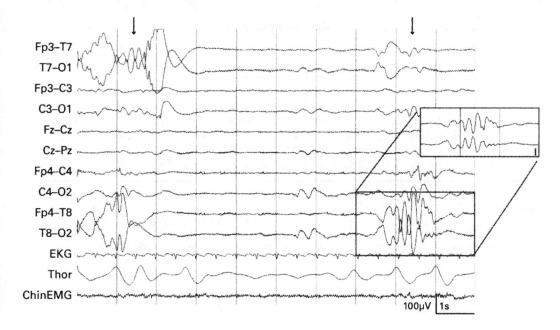

Answers: ECA = 23 weeks + 25 days *(1/7 weeks/day) = 26 4/7 weeks. The background activity is TD, and the findings at the arrows are temporal theta bursts. Both findings indicate developmentally appropriate background activity for ECA.

Discussion: Interpretation of neonatal EEG requires several steps:

1. Calculation of ECA
2. Observation of activity states
3. Recognition of corresponding background activities
4. Identification of physiologic activities upon background activity
5. Determination whether activity states, background activities, and physiologic findings match the stated ECA
6. Identification of pathologic patterns that occur in addition to or instead of expected patterns.

Neonates at ECA <28 weeks have only two discernible activity states: wakefulness and sleep. Activity state is determined through observations of the technologist, review of simultaneous video information (when available), and polygraphic information.

At this early developmental stage, background activities are undifferentiated by state. TD is one of the discontinuous patterns of background EEG of premature neonates. It consists of low-amplitude (<10 μV), mixed activities that are recurrently interrupted by bursts of mixed-frequency activities.

Interburst interval of TD decreases with increasing maturation. At and before 28 weeks ECA, interburst interval is variable and sometimes prolonged up to 90 seconds but usually remains under 40 seconds. Bursts can be asynchronous and asymmetric before 28 weeks, and both properties improve with increasing maturation.

The persistence of TD decreases with maturation. Beyond 28 weeks, sleep begins to differentiate into quiet sleep, with corresponding findings of TD, and active sleep, with corresponding findings of more continuous mixed theta and delta activities. At this stage, activity state and background EEG correspond poorly. In addition, external stimulation does not reliably induce reactive changes in the tracing. A tracing of only unreactive, discontinuous activities after ECA of 30 weeks is a sign of dysmaturity.

The most consistent and earliest appearing of physiologic activities in the premature neonate are *temporal theta bursts* (temporal sawtooth, premature temporal theta). These consist of high-amplitude bursts of epileptiform, rhythmic theta activities occurring in temporal regions. They can occur asynchronously but should be equally persistent bilaterally. The ECA during which they are most frequently observed is 31 weeks, and they become rare beyond 34 weeks.

In this case, activity states limited to sleep and wakefulness, background activities of TD and brief runs of more continuous activities, interburst intervals <40 seconds, poor correspondence between state and EEG, and temporal theta bursts are appropriate for an ECA <28 weeks.

Clinical Pearls

1. TD, bursts of mixed-frequency high-amplitude activities upon suppressed background activities, is present in the earliest neonates.

2. Temporal theta bursts are present in the earliest neonates through approximately ECA of 34 weeks.

3. Unreactive tracings, poor correspondence between activity state and background EEG, and tracings containing solely TD are normal for ECA <28 weeks. More differentiated activity states, background EEG activity, and better correspondence among activity states and EEG should begin by at least ECA of 30 weeks.

REFERENCES

1. Lamblin MD, d'Allest AM, André M, et al: EEG in premature and full-term infants: Developmental features and glossary. Neurophysiol Clin 1999; 29:1232–1219.
2. Werner SS, Stockard JE, Bickford RG: Atlas of Neonatal Electroencephalography. New York, Raven Press, 1977.

PATIENT 24

Premature infant with hypotonia

An EEG is requested in evaluation of hypotonia in an 8-day-old neonate born at 31 4/7 weeks gestational age. The patient is on no sedative medications.

The technologist notes that the patient is asleep and still during this sample. The child is breathing spontaneously. The sample is taken during quiet sleep with background activities of TD.

Questions: What is the estimated conceptional age? Name the findings at electrodes 01/02 *(arrows a)* and at T7 *(arrow b)*. Are these findings normal for this age?

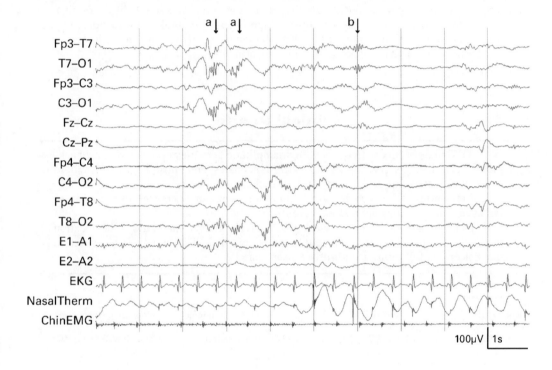

Answers: ECA = 32 5/7 weeks. The findings at 01/02 and T7 are delta brushes, which are normal for premature neonates.

Discussion: With greater maturation, activity states begin to differentiate, and, in turn, activity states become more reliably linked to particularly background EEG activities.

In this nearly ECA 33-week-old neonate, quiet sleep is marked by discontinuous activities, and active sleep and wakefulness begin to be accompanied by continuous activities.

This developmental age marks the peak persistence of physiologic findings termed *delta brushes* (delta waves with superimposed beta activities, beta-delta bursts). Delta brushes are complexes of low-voltage fast activities, usually in the beta or high alpha range, that are superimposed on medium-to-high amplitude delta activities. Their location and association with activity state change with ECA. They initially appear at age 28 weeks in diffuse, multifocal, or central distributions across different states. They are most numerous between 32 and 34 weeks and begin to appear preferentially in temporal or occipital regions during quiet sleep. By the time of their resolution at term, they are confined to occipital regions and to quiet sleep. Note that, in the example, the train of delta brushes is slightly asymmetric. Delta brushes frequently occur asymmetrically and asynchronously.

In this patient, the normal EEG suggested that hypotonia was unlikely to originate from significant cerebral dysfunction. Hypotonia gradually resolved, but its etiology was not identified.

Clinical Pearls

1. TD, bursts of mixed-frequency, high-amplitude activities upon suppressed background activities, is present in the earliest neonates and must begin to yield to continuous patterns of active sleep by at least ECA 30 weeks.

2. Delta brushes are physiologic findings of premature neonates that consist of bursts of beta activities upon slow wave discharges.

3. Delta brushes appear ~28 weeks ECA. With greater maturation, the location gradually becomes limited to occipital regions and their distribution within states to quiet sleep. At full term, delta brushes disappear.

REFERENCES

1. Lamblin MD, d'Allest AM, André M, et al: EEG in premature and full-term infants: Developmental features and glossary. Neurophysiol Clin 1999; 29:1219–1232.
2. Werner SS, Stockard JE, Bickford RG: Atlas of Neonatal Electroencephalography. New York, Raven Press, 1977.

PATIENT 25

Term infant with jitteriness (Part 1)

An EEG is requested to evaluate episodes of jitteriness and oxygen desaturation in a 5-day-old baby born at 37 weeks conceptional age. The infant is on no medications.

The technologist notes that the subject is sleeping during this sample, shown at 30-second and 10-second page lengths.

Questions: What is the ECA? What is the activity state? What is the background activity for this state? What are the sharp transients *(inset)?* Is this EEG normal for a term infant?

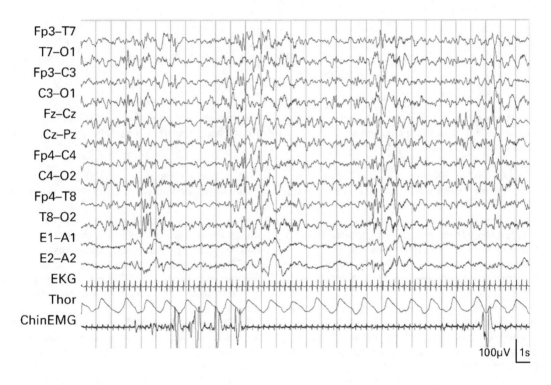

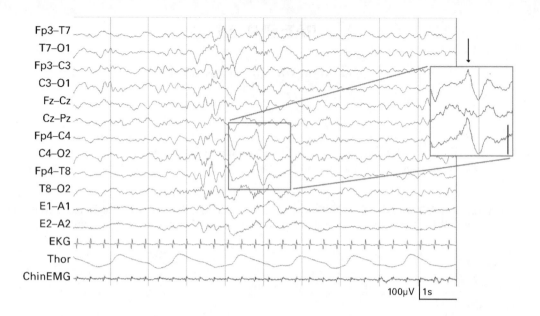

Answers: The ECA is 37 5/7 weeks (term). The activity state is quiet sleep, and the background activity is TA. The sharp transients in the inset are frontal sharp transients (encoche frontale). This EEG is normal for a term infant.

Discussion: Starting at >28 weeks and progressing through 36 weeks, neonates develop stable and clear activity states of wakefulness, active sleep, and quiet sleep.

Quiet sleep is the precursor to non-REM sleep. On polygraphic channels, eyes are closed and movements sparse, breathing is regular and rhythmic, tone is relatively low, and most movements cease.

One of the main background activities of quiet sleep in the term neonate is TA. TA is a discontinuous pattern of sleep in which slower, lower-amplitude background activities (1–5 cps) alternate with bursts of mixed faster- and higher-amplitude activities. The bursts appear roughly every 4–8 seconds and last 2–5 seconds.

TA usually emerges by 36–38 weeks ECA. TA is the last discontinuous pattern that persists in the term infant. Continuous activities of non-REM sleep begin to replace TA as development proceeds, a process that continues through the first several months of life.

TA must be distinguished from other discontinuous patterns, such as dysmature TD or frank burst-suppression. In comparison to TD, activities between bursts in TA consist of ongoing delta or theta activities with amplitudes exceeding 10 μV, whereas bursts in TD occur upon activities that are typically <10 μV. Normal TA appears as just one of two or more patterns during the hour of the neonatal tracing. Burst-suppression, on the other hand, may be unreactive to stimulation or remain invariant throughout the recording. Other physiologic findings appropriate to ECA, such as delta brushes or encoche frontale, appear in concert with TA and may be present in dysmature TD, whereas they are absent in burst-suppression.

The tracings of normal premature and term neonates also display various sharp transients. *Encoches frontales* (French for frontal notches, frontal sharp transients) are biphasic, high-amplitude sharp transients that initially appear ~34 weeks ECA, are most frequent at 36 weeks, and taper in incidence through term. They can be unilateral or bilateral but have equal persistence bilaterally. Sometimes encoches frontales occur in brief runs and may appear with less sharp morphologies, leading to a pattern called *anterior dysrhythmia.*

Various epileptiform transients, especially predominant in frontal and temporal regions, appear preferentially during bursts of discontinuous activities. Focal spikes that persist through different sleep-wake stages may indicate abnormalities.

Clinical Pearls

1. Term infants have three activity states: wakefulness, active sleep, and quiet sleep.

2. TA is the last discontinuous pattern to persist in the term infant. It begins to appear approximately at ECA of 36 weeks and begins to evolve to continuous non-REM sleep after birth.

3. Encoches frontales are normal high-amplitude, often asynchronous, biphasic sharp transients that emerge around 34 weeks, peak at 36 weeks, and resolve through postpartum development.

REFERENCES

1. Lamblin MD, d'Allest AM, André M, et al: EEG in premature and full-term infants: Developmental features and glossary. Neurophysiol Clin 1999; 29:1219–1232.
2. Werner SS, Stockard JE, Bickford RG: Atlas of Neonatal Electroencephalography. New York, Raven Press, 1977.

PATIENT 26

Term infant with jitteriness (Part 2)

This is another sample from the ECA 37 5/7 week neonate from the previous case, recorded just before the period of TA.

The subject is sleeping during this sample, shown at 30-second and 10-second page lengths.

Questions: What is the activity state? What is the background activity for this state?

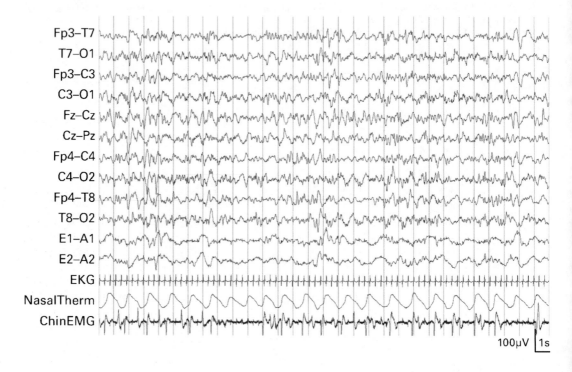

100μV 1s

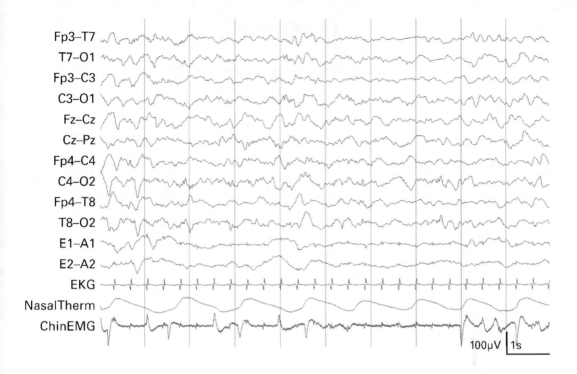

Fp3–T7
T7–O1
Fp3–C3
C3–O1
Fz–Cz
Cz–Pz
Fp4–C4
C4–O2
Fp4–T8
T8–O2
E1–A1
E2–A2
EKG
NasalTherm
ChinEMG

100µV 1s

Answers: The activity state is quiet sleep. The background activity is high-voltage slowing.

Discussion: Quiet sleep in term infants can be accompanied by two types of background activities. One is TA, seen in the previous example. The other background activity is denoted by *high voltage slowing (HVS)*. HVS is a continuous pattern of 50–150 µV, diffusely distributed, semi-rhythmic delta activities that emerges in the term infant. HVS typically precedes the onset of TA. Stimulation during TA can provoke HVS. With further maturation, the duration of HVS in quiet sleep increases and the persistence of TA declines. HVS can be thought of as the morphologic precursor to non-REM, slow wave sleep.

Transitions between HVS and TA may be difficult to clearly mark, as the overall amplitude of activities during this sample wax and wane in an alternating pattern, as visible on the 30-second page lengths.

Clinical Pearls

1. HVS is a continuous pattern of quiet sleep that emerges at term.
2. HVS usually precedes a period of TA.
3. HVS and increasing duration of bursts in TA gradually form more mature non-REM sleep in the postnatal, term infant.

REFERENCES
1. Lamblin MD, d'Allest AM, André M, et al: EEG in premature and full-term infants: Developmental features and glossary. Neurophysiol Clin 1999; 29:1219–1232.
2. Werner SS, Stockard JE, Bickford RG: Atlas of Neonatal Electroencephalography. New York, Raven Press, 1977.

PATIENT 27

Term infant with jitteriness (Part 3)

This is a third sample from the normal-term neonate from the previous cases, recorded 15 minutes after the period of TA.

The subject is sleeping during this sample, shown at 30-second and 10-second page lengths.

Questions: Identify the source of potentials in EOG channels *(arrows)* and the activity state. What is the background activity?

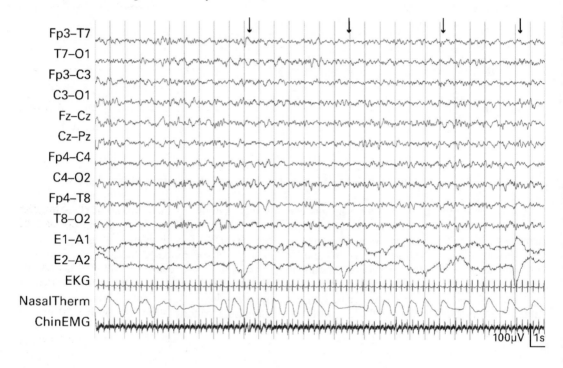

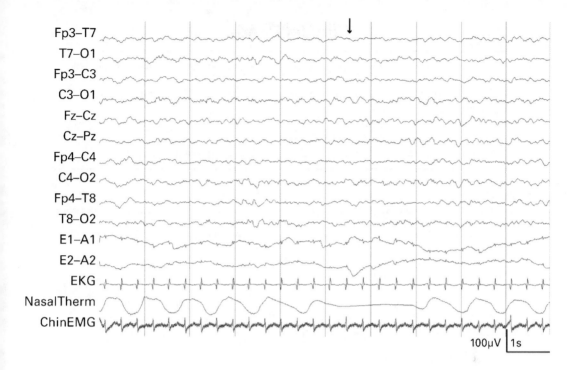

Answers: The source of potentials in EOG channels *(arrows)* is eye movements, specifically REMs, and the activity state is active sleep, defined by REMs, relatively low EMG activity, irregular breathing patterns, and technologist's observations of sleep. The background activity consists of continuous, low- to medium-amplitude mixed frequency activities.

Discussion: Differentiation in activity states begins at ECA >28 weeks. *Active sleep* is the immature precursor to REM sleep. Active sleep is identified by the technologist's observations of eye closure and paroxysmal activities, such as facial grimacing or finger posturing. EOG records phasic eye movements. Respiratory monitoring shows irregular breathing patterns or brief apneas. EMG may show relative hypotonia.

Full-term neonates spend about 50% of a recording in active sleep. Whereas children and adults begin sleep with non-REM sleep, neonates start in active sleep. As the infant matures, the persistence of active sleep decreases. Eventually, REM occupies approximately 25% of adult nocturnal sleep.

The EEG of early active sleep consists of continuous activities, a pattern of mixed, low-amplitude (~25 µV) theta and delta activities. Continuous activities of active sleep in term neonates are differentiated into two types: a low-amplitude (~25 µV), irregular pattern of mixed theta and alpha frequencies that typically appear before an episode of quiet sleep, and a higher-amplitude pattern of semirhythmic higher-amplitude (~25–50 µV) delta activities with intermixed theta activities that appear after quiet sleep. Terminology differs among authors. Synonyms for the mainly lower-amplitude, faster-frequency pattern are *low-voltage irregular* pattern (LVI) and *activité moyenne* (French for average or mixed frequencies). The pattern of higher-amplitude, predominantly delta activity, is usually termed *mixed frequency* or *continuous activities*. Simple description of activities accompanying active sleep is the clearest way out of confusing terminology and is the robust method relied on during this review.

In the present case, active sleep is accompanied by continuous EEG activities of 25–30 µV, predominantly delta activities with occasional theta activities.

Clinical Pearls

1. Active sleep comprises approximately 50% of the normal full-term neonatal tracing.

2. The healthy neonate transitions from one to another activity state at least once during an hour's recording.

3. Active sleep is identified by the appearance of sleep, phasic eye movements, hypotonia, and ongoing phasic patient activities.

4. Continuous, mixed frequency EEG activities accompany active sleep.

REFERENCES

1. Lamblin MD, d'Allest AM, André M, et al: EEG in premature and full-term infants: Developmental features and glossary. Neurophysiol Clin 1999; 29:1219–1232.
2. Werner SS, Stockard JE, Bickford RG: Atlas of Neonatal Electroencephalography. New York, Raven Press, 1977.

PATIENT 28

A 6-week-old term infant with spells

Parents of a 6-week-old infant born at gestational age 35 weeks note that their son has spells of stiffening.

The technologist notes that the subject is opening and closing his eyes spontaneously during the time from which the sample is taken.

Questions: Identify the activity state. What is the background activity?

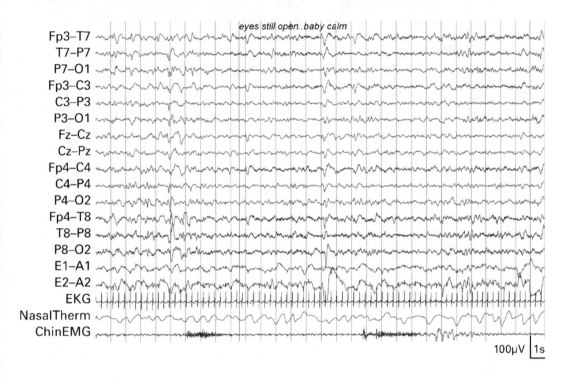

Answers: Spontaneous eye opening denotes wakefulness. The background activity consists of continuous, low-to-medium amplitude mixed-frequency activities.

Discussion: The activity state of wakefulness is difficult to distinguish from active sleep in many neonates. The most reliable sign is technologist's observations of spontaneous eye opening. Restlessness or agitation, irregular breathing patterns, and other phasic movements may also be present on polygraphy.

The EEG of wakefulness consists of continuous, rather featureless, mixed-frequency activities.

Clinical Pearls

1. Wakefulness is most reliably determined by observation of spontaneous eye opening. Restlessness or agitation and irregular breathing are other evidence of wakefulness.
2. Continuous, mixed-frequency EEG activities accompany wakefulness.

REFERENCES

1. Lamblin MD, d'Allest AM, André M, et al: EEG in premature and full-term infants: Developmental features and glossary. Neurophysiol Clin 1999; 29:1219–1232.
2. Werner SS, Stockard JE, Bickford RG: Atlas of Neonatal Electroencephalography. New York, Raven Press, 1977.

PATIENT 29

Term infant with apnea

An EEG is requested to determine the cause of recurrent apneas without bradycardia in an 8-day-old infant who was born at age 39 weeks estimated gestational age. The infant had movements thought to be seizures on the day of birth. An intraventricular hemorrhage is found. The patient is on phenobarbital.

The technologist notes that the patient is on a ventilator and is unarousable. Both 30-second and 10-second page lengths are shown in the following.

Questions: What is the ECA? Identify the activity state and background activity. Is the background activity appropriate for ECA?

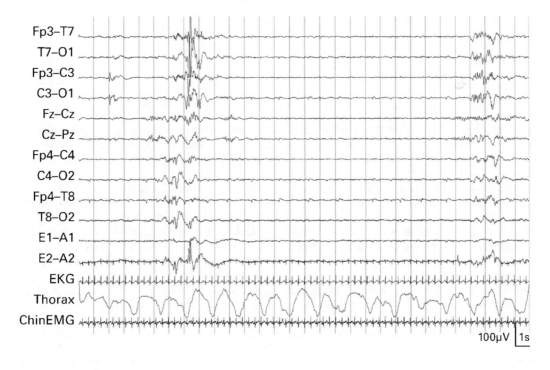

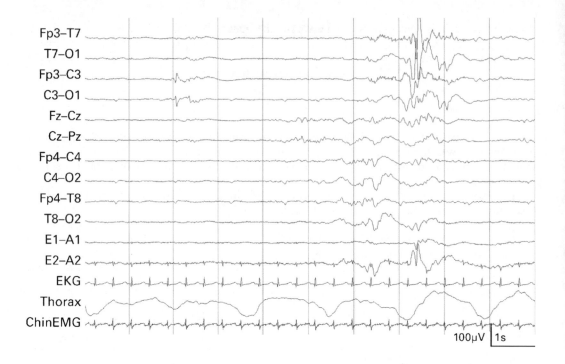

Fp3–T7				
T7–O1				
Fp3–C3				
C3–O1				
Fz–Cz				
Cz–Pz				
Fp4–C4				
C4–O2				
Fp4–T8				
T8–O2				
E1–A1				
E2–A2				
EKG				
Thorax				
ChinEMG				

100µV 1s

Answers: The ECA is 40 1/7 weeks. The activity state is indeterminate sleep versus comatose. Note that the breathing pattern is unreliably regular from mechanical ventilation. The background activity is suppression-burst. This activity is inappropriate for the ECA.

Discussion: As seen in earlier examples, TD is a premature pattern identified by bursts of activity that interrupt relatively suppressed activities. It may be difficult to tell the difference between TD and suppression-burst. Suppression-burst is distinguished from TD by the former's lack of reactivity, the lack of normal physiologic findings, such as temporal theta bursts or delta brushes, and the lack of transitions to other activity states.

Rather than focus on qualitative differences, some investigators link the duration of the inter-burst interval to prognosis. Interburst intervals decrease with increasing ECA. Below 30 weeks, interburst intervals up to 40 seconds are appropriate. At 36 weeks, the latest ECA during which TD is appropriate, interburst interval typically is <10 seconds. An interburst interval >30 seconds during discontinuous activities in term infants correlates with both unfavorable neurologic outcome and subsequent epilepsy. Electrocerebral silence (ECS)—the total absence of cerebral activity, and, by extension, a pattern with an "extremely long" interburst interval—indicates severe encephalopathy and poor prognosis. Although ECS is evidence that supports the diagnosis of brain death in adults, such an electrographic

diagnosis cannot be made in infants. Nevertheless, ECS is an extremely unfavorable finding in the premature or term infant.

Despite the implications of poor prognosis in these patterns in neonates, prognosis cannot be reliably determined from a single tracing. Certainly, unremitting suppression-burst is a poor prognostic finding, but its appearance and subsequent correction within a short period of time (~24 hours) have little prognostic value. As with older patients, suppression-burst is a non-specific pattern that may result from reversible causes (phenobarbital, for example) or from dire causes (prolonged hypoxia).

In the present case, the abnormal background activity supports a diagnosis of encephalopathy. Because the baby was ventilated, no apneic events occurred, so the tracing cannot directly determine their cause. Two factors, however, provide evidence that the apneic events probably represent epileptic seizures. First, some investigators have demonstrated that abnormal background activity on a routine tracing in neonates who are at risk for seizures predicts their occurrence within the subsequent 18–24 hours (with 96% sensitivity and 80% specificity). Second, the clinical information that apneic events occurred without bradycardia is consistent with an epileptic cause; traditionally, nonepileptic apnea is associated with reflex bradycardia. Therefore, the abnormal EEG and absence of bradycardia suggest that seizures are a likely etiology of apnea.

Clinical Pearls

1. Interburst intervals of discontinuous activity gradually decrease with increasing ECA in the healthy neonates.
2. Prolonged interburst intervals in discontinuous activities are predictive of poor neurologic outcome on serial recordings.
3. Abnormal background activity in neonates who have illnesses predisposing to present as seizures often predicts the occurrence of subsequent seizures.

REFERENCES

1. Fenichel GM, Olson BJ, Fitzpatrick JE: Heart rate changes in convulsive and nonconvulsive neonatal apnea. Ann Neurol 1980; 7(6):577–582.
2. Hahn J, Monyer H, Tharp B: Interburst interval measurements in the EEGs of premature infants with normal neurological outcome. Electroencephalogr Clin Neurophysiol 1989; 73:410–418.
3. Laroia N, Guillet R, Burchfiel J, McBride MC: EEG background as predictor of electrographic seizures in high-risk neonates. Epilepsia 1998; 39:545–551.
4. Menache C, Bourgeois B, Volpe J: Prognostic value of neonatal discontinuous EEG. Pediatr Neurol 2002; 27:93–101.
5. Okumura A, Hayakawa F, Kato T, et al: Developmental outcome and types of chronic-stage EEG abnormalities in preterm infants. Dev Med Child Neurol 2002; 44:729–734.

PATIENT 30

Term infant with encephalitis and seizures

An EEG is requested to determine the cause of clonic limb movements in an 8-day-old girl (gestational age = 39 weeks) who has bilateral intraventricular hemorrhages and herpetic encephalitis. She is treated with phenobarbital, acyclovir, and antibiotics.

The technologist notes that the patient is occasionally arousable and mechanically ventilated. For a portion of the tracing not pictured, continuous activities of active sleep are recorded. These 30- and 10-second samples are taken 10 minutes before active sleep.

Questions: What is the ECA? Identify the activity state and accompanying background activity. Is background activity appropriate for the ECA? Of sharp transients marked *a, b,* or *c,* which are physiologic and which are pathologic?

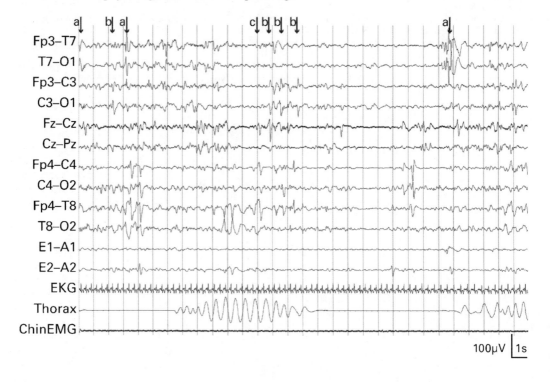

100µV | 1s

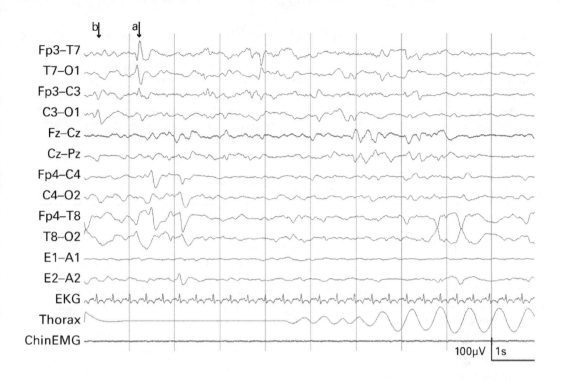

Answers: The ECA is 40 1/7 weeks. The activity state and background activity are most consistent with quiet sleep and TD. Note that the breathing pattern is unreliably regular from mechanical ventilation. This activity is inappropriate for the ECA. Pathologic monophasic and polyphasic high-amplitude left temporal spikes and sharp waves (*arrows a*) and independent left central spikes and sharp waves of both negative and positive polarity (*arrows b*) occurred most frequently. Right temporal sharp waves and broader-based sharp transients and right central spikes also appear in the sample. Physiologic encoches frontales were also present (*arrow c*).

Discussion: *Dysmaturity*—the persistence of a pattern consistent with an earlier developmental stage—is an important abnormality in the neonatal tracing. The delayed persistence of a pattern of more than 2 weeks is a reasonable boundary beyond which a pattern should be considered dysmature. For example, continuous patterns are expected to emerge after ECA 28 weeks; therefore, the lack of continuous activities in a >30-week-old neonate implies encephalopathy. Similarly, the persistence of TD > ECA 36 weeks + 2 weeks, as in the present case, is abnormal. Findings from the whole tracing, not just that confined to the previous sample, are required to distinguish between persistent TD and suppression-burst. This case was interpreted as dysmature TD rather than suppression-burst because of continuous activities seen in the latter portion of the recording.

Background activities provide the best prognostic information, but other abnormal findings help. Multifocal and frequent spikes, such as those shown in the current case, are abnormal.

Focal sharp waves and spikes present unique problems in neonatal tracings. Although spikes and sharp waves are defined with the same criteria among neonates, children, and adults, the types of epileptiform discharges and their significance differ.

Spikes seen in children and adults typically have negative potentials recorded at the scalp, whereas neonatal spikes may have positive potentials. Usually, polarity of neonatal spikes has no special association with pathology. Two exceptions are *Rolandic positive spikes* (positive central sharp waves) and midtemporal positive spikes; these may be found in intraventricular hemorrhage. The present consensus, however, is that these discharges are not specific for hemorrhage but can also be present in other deep white matter lesions.

Another difference between spikes seen in neonates and those seen in older subjects is that the former are not specific to epilepsy. Neonatal spikes are a nonspecific indicator of focal pathology or diffuse encephalopathy.

Spikes are commonly seen in normal neonates, especially during bursts of TD in the premature neonate and within quiet sleep and TA in full-term neonates. Frontal sharp transients (encoche frontale), for example, are normal despite their epileptiform morphology.

Unfortunately, no clear guidelines separate normal from abnormal spikes in neonates. Spikes tend to be abnormal, if they occur in rhythmic runs, if they occur in one location only, if they recur within the low-amplitude portions of discontinuous patterns, if they persist through continuous background activities, or have a polyphasic morphology. In this case, most spikes occurred within the high-amplitude bursts of TD, but others occurred in between.

Clinical Pearls

1. Persistent TD in the full-term infant is evidence of dysmaturity.

2. Spikes can be normal in the premature and full-term infant and are most evident within bursts of discontinuous background patterns.

3. Abnormal spikes tend to recur in trains, appear unilaterally, occur in between bursts of discontinuous patterns, and persist during continuous patterns.

4. Positive central and positive midtemporal sharp waves may indicate deep white matter lesions, but other pathologic spikes have more association with nonspecific diffuse or focal abnormalities and do not necessarily predict higher risk of subsequent seizures.

REFERENCES

1. Hahn J, Monyer H, Tharp B: Interburst interval measurements in the EEGs of premature infants with normal neurological outcome. Electroencephalogr Clin Neurophysiol 1989; 73:410–418.
2. Menache C, Bourgeois B, Volpe J: Prognostic value of neonatal discontinuous EEG. Pediatr Neurol 2002; 27:93–101.
3. Okumura A, Hayakawa F, Kato T, et al: Developmental outcome and types of chronic-stage EEG abnormalities in preterm infants. Dev Med Child Neurol 2002; 44:729–734.

PATIENT 31

A 7-year-old boy with nocturnal seizures

An EEG is requested in evaluation of nocturnal seizures that consisted of speech difficulties and right lower facial movements in a 7-year-old, otherwise healthy, boy whose father had childhood-onset seizures that resolved.

The patient takes no medications. Although awake in this segment, spikes were much more frequent with drowsiness (*arrows*). The sample is shown in both bipolar and referential montages.

Questions: What is the location of the negative-polarity spike discharges? What polarity (negative or positive) is displayed at electrode F3 (best seen at *arrow a*)? What epilepsy syndrome best fits the clinical description and electrographic findings?

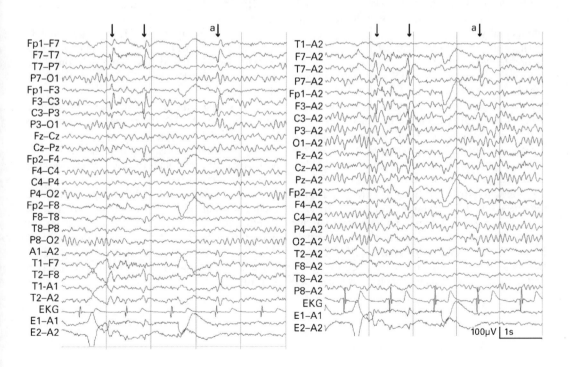

Answers: Frequent negative-polarity spikes are present in left centrotemporal regions. A positive polarity, defining a horizontal dipole, can be seen in the left frontal region. The syndrome pictured here is benign childhood epilepsy with centrotemporal spikes (Rolandic epilepsy).

Discussion: Benign childhood epilepsy with centrotemporal spikes (BECTS), also known as benign centrotemporal lobe epilepsy of childhood and benign Rolandic epilepsy, is classified as an idiopathic, localization-related epilepsy.

Ages of onset range between 3 and 13 years, but most cases occur between ages 5 and 10. BECTS is one of the more common forms of childhood epilepsy. The most important clinical characteristic of BECTS is that it resolves spontaneously in most patients by ages 13–14. Its recognition, therefore, is important to prevent overtreatment and to provide an excellent prognosis to worried families.

BECTS features simple partial seizures that involve facial muscles, thus preventing speech and frequently causing drooling. Many patients describe sensations of "electricity" or other paresthesia of the tongue and lower face. Although most episodes are brief, some patients experience secondary generalization in a typical "Jacksonian march" of spread of motor activity to an upper and then a lower limb. Most seizures occur during sleep, so seizures tend to occur nocturnally or during naps. Patients are neurologically and intellectually normal.

The EEG can distinguish BECTS from less favorable syndromes.

Location. Spikes in BECTS are located in centrotemporal regions. About 60% of subjects have spikes confined to one side, but 40% have independent bilateral or even multifocal spikes.

Polarity. Spikes in BECTS usually feature a *horizontal dipole*. In the previous example, the discharge has maximum negativity in the left centrotemporal region and projects anteriorly and medially to a positivity in the left frontal region. As in this example, dipoles in BECTS usually appear ipsilateral, medial, and anterior to the affected centrotemporal region. A dipole in BECTS results from the location of the epileptic focus in the primary motor cortex deep within the central (Rolandic) sulcus. A horizontal orientation allows the capture of the positive part of the electrical potential. In contrast, most other IEDs have negative potentials that project perpendicularly; the downwardly directed positivities project to a region without electrodes.

A dipole may be difficult to identify on longitudinal bipolar montages because the amplitude of the positivity may be overwhelmed, both visually and electrically, by the high amplitude of the negative discharge. Dipoles, however, can be often picked up by viewing Rolandic spikes with a referential montage referenced to the contralateral ear. A phase reversal in the referential montage indicates an electric dipole, if the reference electrode is not *contaminated* (located within the electrical field of the discharge).

Morphology. IEDs of BECTS are high amplitude, often 150–250 μV. Spikes, although epileptiform, are often somewhat blunted in comparison to IEDs seen in other syndromes. Many spikes in BECTS could be better termed *sharp waves* because the high amplitudes often create baseline durations >70 milliseconds. IEDs in BECTS also feature prominent after-slow potentials.

Activation. IEDs in BECTS are activated by drowsiness and light sleep. Patients with suspected BECTS should have an EEG containing these states if the waking EEG contains no abnormalities.

In this case, the EEG findings and clinical picture of BECTS led the requesting neurologist to manage the patient by "expectant observation"; in other words, the patient received no anticonvulsant medications and was not subjected to further testing. Anticonvulsant treatment is optional and depends on the further incidence and severity of seizures as well as parental and patient preferences. A seizure-free period of 1–2 years, along with a follow-up EEG that documents resolution of Rolandic spikes, is the usual approach to discontinuing anticonvulsant medications.

Clinical Pearls

1. Rolandic spikes are high-amplitude, centrotemporal, blunted spikes with prominent slow afterpotentials. A dipole anterior and transverse to centrotemporal regions is frequently present.

2. Benign childhood epilepsy with centrotemporal spikes is a benign idiopathic localization-related epilepsy syndrome marked by childhood onset, sleep-associated simple partial seizures, normal intellect, and excellent prognosis.

3. Dipoles of IEDs in BECTS are most easily recognized in referential montages. Phase reversal in referential montages indicates either a contaminated reference or an electrical dipole.

REFERENCES

1. Loiseau P, Duche B, Cordova S, et al: Prognosis of benign childhood epilepsy with centro-temporal spikes: A follow-up of 168 patients. Epilepsia 1988; 29:229–235.
2. Murphy JV, Dehkharghani F: Diagnosis of childhood seizure disorders. Epilepsia 1994; 35:S7–S17.

PATIENT 32

An 11-year-old boy with nocturnal hemiconvulsions and visual seizures

An 11-year-old boy presents for evaluation of several episodes of nocturnal convulsions that cause leftward eye deviation and right arm and leg clonus. Although most episodes occur at night during sleep, some rare episodes are preceded by brief, poorly formed visual hallucinations of colored spots and visual distortion. Headaches and nausea follow most events, and migraines have been problematic for several years.

The recordings are performed with the patient awake, and samples are shown in both bipolar and referential montages. He takes carbamazepine.

Questions: Identify the location and polarity of spikes in this sample (*arrows*). What epilepsy syndrome does the tracing suggest for this clinical presentation?

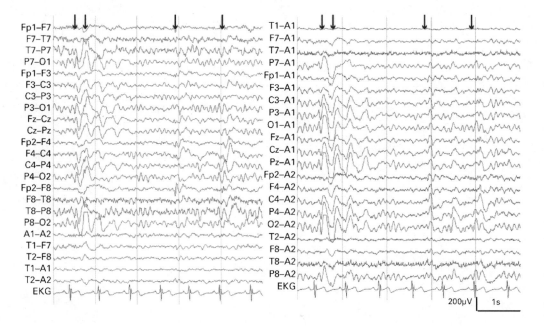

Answers: The arrows indicate bioccipital spikes with maximum negativity at the end of the longitudinal chain. A burst of occipitally dominant rhythmic delta activity is present. An irregular train of more poorly shaped occipital sharp transients occurs afterward. This tracing suggests a diagnosis of benign occipital epilepsy of childhood.

Discussion: Benign occipital epilepsy of childhood (BOEC), also known as childhood epilepsy with occipital paroxysms, is an idiopathic, localization-related epilepsy syndrome that is sometimes difficult to distinguish because of controversy in its gathering or separation of subtypes.

Most authorities acknowledge two subtypes of BOEC based on age of onset. The early subtype has ages of onset between 3 and 5 years; the late subtype has its onset between ages 7 and 10. Seizures in BOEC usually feature positive visual symptoms, such as scotomata, fortifications, or hallucinations, or negative symptoms, such as amaurosis. Convulsions usually occur during sleep and range from versive seizures marked by forced lateral eye deviation and body turning to hemiconvulsions.

Seizures are often followed by migraine-like headaches with typical symptoms of nausea and malaise. Younger patients tend to experience more migraine-like symptoms, such as nausea, whereas older patients typically complain more of visual symptoms. BOEC is seen more often in girls than boys. The seizures of BOEC usually resolve by adolescence and are associated with normal intellectual development.

Both syndrome subtypes feature similar EEG findings.

Location. Spikes occur symmetrically in bioccipital regions. Occipital spikes can be difficult to recognize because readers become used to upward-pointing spikes. Occipital spikes, however, point down at the end of a bipolar chain because the negative potential makes G1 of the posterior channel less negative than G2, leading to a downward deflection. An aid to confirm the identity of putative occipital spikes is to reverse the inputs to the channel so that transients point up in a more familiar direction (on paper EEG, accomplished by viewing transients through the back of the page and upside down), as shown here:

The same effect can usually be produced by viewing the findings with the use of a referential montage. Such maneuvers are often necessary to distinguish occipital spikes from the normal slowing and sharp transients that dwell in posterior regions.

Activation. Occipital spikes usually appear in bursts (occipital paroxysms) and are activated during eye closure and attenuated by eye opening.

Other syndromes also present with occipital spikes. Idiopathic photosensitive epilepsies, for example, differ from BOEC in that seizures are triggered by flashing lights from sources ranging from computer screens, video games, or flashing sunlight in a moving car. Occipital or generalized spikes are provoked in the laboratory by photic stimulation.

Occipital spikes are sometimes seen in childhood migraine. It is particularly confusing because of the association of migraine-like headaches and visual fortifications that are often present in both migraine and BOEC.

Symptomatic partial epilepsy caused by epileptic lesions of the occipital region can also present with occipital spikes. Spikes from symptomatic lesions, however, often do not display changing persistence with eye opening or closure, are usually asymmetric, can have field or maximum negativity extending beyond occipital regions, and may appear with focal slowing. Finally, a possibly overlapping benign epilepsy, Panayiotopoulos syndrome, characterized by autonomic seizures (gastrointestinal symptoms, pallor, and ictal syncope) may have occipital spikes, but is also associated with high rates of multifocal spikes or even generalized spikes. Ongoing debate is attempting to clarify divisions between BOEC and other epilepsies that commonly feature occipital spikes.

P4–O2 ⋯⋯ O2–P4 ⋯⋯ spike ↓ / ↑ spike

Clinical Pearls

1. BOEC is a benign childhood epilepsy marked by two ages of onset.

2. BOEC must be distinguished from symptomatic localization-related epilepsies that originate from occipital lesions. Symmetry, activation with eye closure, and lack of focal slowing argue against a symptomatic epilepsy.

3. Identification of occipital spikes can be facilitated by reversing channel inputs.

REFERENCES

1. Gastaut H: Benign epilepsy of childhood with occipital paroxysms. In Roger J, Dravet C, Bureau F (eds): Epileptic Syndromes in Infancy, Childhood and Adolescence. London, John Libby, 1985, pp 170–179.
2. Panayiotopoulos CP: Benign childhood epileptic syndromes with occipital spikes: New classification proposed by the International League Against Epilepsy. J Child Neurol 2000; 15(8): 548–552.

PATIENT 33

A 21-year-old woman with occipital sharp transients during sleep

An EEG following sleep deprivation is requested for a 21-year-old woman with recent spells of confusion and dissociation. Her spells do not respond to lamotrigine.

The sample is taken from sleep.

Questions: In what sleep stage is the patient? Identify the location and polarity of the discharges under the bar. What is the clinical significance of these discharges?

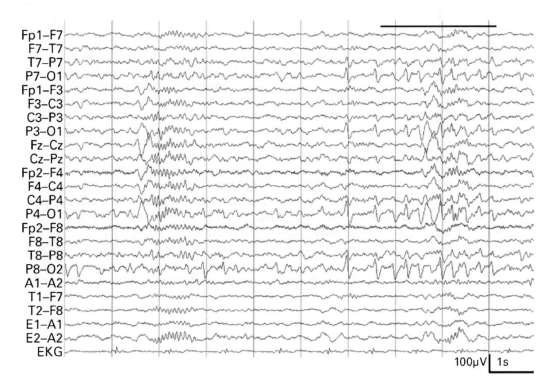

Answers: The patient is in stage 2 sleep, as identified by sleep spindles. The discharges under the bar are occipital sharp transients, with positive polarity. *Positive occipital sharp transients of sleep (POSTS) are normal findings of sleep.*

Discussion: POSTS are a normal finding of light sleep, especially in youthful subjects.

Location: They occur bioccipitally and synchronously but may not be symmetric in amplitude.

Polarity and morphology: POSTS are positive in potential, λ-shaped (sometimes termed "checkmark-shaped"), and usually biphasic, with an initial prominent positivity followed by a negative, broader potential. They typically occur in trains.

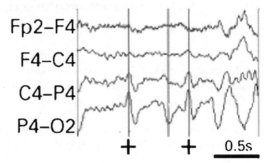

The POSTS in this example are particularly prominent and sharp, making them easily confused with occipital IEDs. Their identification is made easier by keeping in mind the behavior of focal discharges at the end of a bipolar chain.

In this excerpt, the positive potential beyond O2 makes the G1 input of channel P4-O2 less positive than the G2 input. According to the pen rule, the pen points up because the G1 input is relatively more negative than G2. Similarly, the positive potential at C4-P4 causes a slightly smaller upswing of the pen because the potential is further away.

Clinical Pearls

1. POSTS are positive sharp transients seen at the occiput, frequently occurring in trains; they may appear during light sleep.

2. Distinction between pathologic occipital IEDs and normal POSTS requires recognition of polarity.

PATIENT 34

A 54-year-old woman with medically intractable complex partial seizures

A 54-year-old woman has medically intractable complex partial seizures consisting of speech arrest, confusion, chewing, and hand movements, usually preceded by an aura of gastrointestinal "lifting." She had severe febrile convulsions as an infant, and unprovoked seizures began at age 14.

This tracing is a baseline prior to intensive video-EEG monitoring in consideration of epilepsy surgery. The patient is taking levetiracetam.

The sample is shown in both bipolar and longitudinal montages during wakefulness.

Questions: In what location are the spikes (*arrows*)? What other abnormalities in the same location are present? With which epilepsy syndrome is this case most consistent?

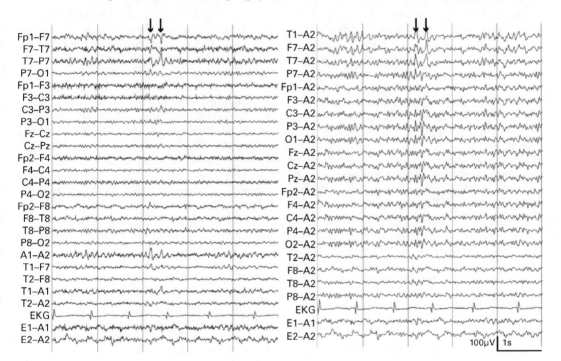

Answers: The arrows indicate spikes and sharp waves with maximum negativity at the anterior temporal region. They are frequent and appear with slowing in the theta range. The syndrome of prodromal, infantile injury, emergence during adolescence of complex partial seizures with auras after a latent period, and medical intractability is most consistent with *mesial temporal lobe epilepsy* (MTLE).

Discussion: MTLE is the most frequent syndrome associated with medically intractable epilepsy in adults. It is a symptomatic, localization-related epilepsy syndrome defined by several key clinical and electrographic features.

Many patients have a history of infantile injury to the central nervous system. Injuries associated with MTLE are atypical febrile convulsions, meningoencephalitis, or significant head trauma. Many patients experience a latent period through early childhood with emergence of seizures near puberty or later.

Patients with MTLE usually have complex partial seizures with or without secondary generalization. Early studies refer to "psychomotor seizures" because of the involvement of brain regions mediating autonomic regulation, affect, memory, and sensorimotor association functions. Most patients experience *auras*, warning events, that, despite their epileptic origin, may show no abnormalities during their occurrence on scalp recordings.

The lesion found in MTLE is *hippocampal sclerosis*, which involves selective neuronal loss and gliosis of the hippocampus, amygdala, and mammillary bodies. Widespread limbic involvement leads some to use the more general terms *mesial sclerosis* and *limbic epilepsy*. The MRI in MTLE usually shows unilateral hippocampal atrophy in T1-weighted sequences and sclerosis (high intensity) in T2-weighted and *fluid-attenuation inversion recovery* (FLAIR) sequences. About 25% of subjects have bilateral atrophy with one side worse.

The EEG findings in this case are typical for MTLE.

Location. Sharp waves and spikes in MTLE usually appear in the anterior temporal region, demonstrated here with phase reversal at F7 in the bipolar montage and equal amplitudes at F7, T1, and T7 in the referential montage. IEDs in MTLE often have a characteristic "basal" location, with maximum negativity present in anterior or true temporal electrodes and an electrical field visible in the contralateral temporal region.

Polarity and morphology. In contrast to Rolandic spikes seen in BECTS, IEDs in MTLE appear with maximum negativity more inferiorly and anteriorly and lack a dipole.

Activation and reactivity. Although IEDs in MTLE can be activated by sleep or sleep deprivation, activation is less profound than that seen in BECTS. Well-defined cerebral fields, after slow potentials, and epileptiform morphology with durations between 70 and 200 μV define these potentials as epileptogenic sharp waves rather than benign interictal epileptiform discharges.

IEDs are found in about two-thirds of patients with MTLE during routine recording. Prolonged recording (mean duration 7 days in one study) increases sensitivity of IEDs to 80%. Because one-third of patients with MTLE may have independent, bitemporal IEDs, the specificity of interictal spikes in the determination of the side of onset of epileptic seizures in MTLE is controversial.

In addition to left anterior midtemporal sharp waves, this particular recording also features arrhythmic theta activity in the same distribution as the sharp waves. The finding indicates that the underlying brain has a nonspecific neuronal dysfunction (a physiologic lesion) or a structural lesion. Its appearance with IEDs indicates a neuronal abnormality that is potentially epileptogenic.

Clinical Pearls

1. Mesial temporal lobe epilepsy is the most common syndrome of medically intractable epilepsy in adults and consists of complex partial seizures with and without secondary generalization—usually a history of antecedent injury and latent onset, MRI findings of hippocampal sclerosis, and interictal EEG showing anterior temporal sharp waves or spike discharges, with or without focal slowing.

2. The sensitivity of a single, routine EEG in yielding IEDs in known epileptics is greater than 50%. Repeat routine recordings yield up to about 80% after the third recording.

REFERENCES

1. Annegers J, Hauser W, Shirts S, Kurland L: Factors prognostic of unprovoked seizures after febrile convulsions. N Engl J Med 1987; 316(9): 493–498.
2. Cascino GD, Trenerry MR, So EL, et al: Routine EEG and temporal lobe epilepsy: Relation to long-term EEG monitoring, quantitative MRI, and operative outcome. Epilepsia 1996; 37(7): 651–656.
3. Mathern G, Babb T, Armstrong D: Hippocampal sclerosis. In Engel JJ, Pedley T (eds): Epilepsy: A Comprehensive Textbook. New York, Raven Press, 1997, pp 133–155.
4. Walczak TS, Radtke RA, McNamara JO, et al: Anterior temporal lobectomy for complex partial seizures: Evaluation, results, and long-term follow-up in 100 cases. Neurology 1990; 40:413–418.

PATIENT 35

A 56-year-old drowsy man with visual hallucinations

An EEG is requested to evaluate spells of hallucinations in a 56-year-old man taking simvastatin. The recording is performed with the patient drowsy.

Questions: Identify the sharp waves (*bar a*) and their clinical significance. Identify the periodic sharp waves (*arrowheads b*).

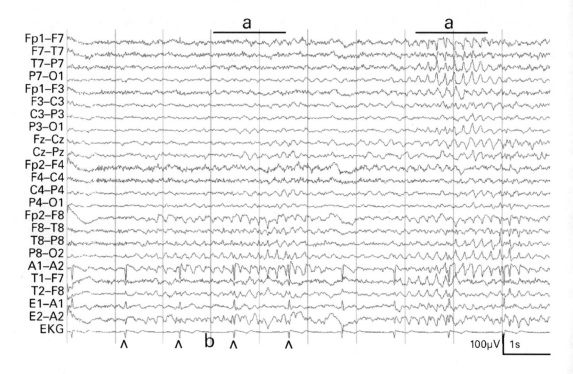

Focal Sharp Transients and Localization-Related Epilepsy

Answers: During drowsiness, there are runs of rhythmic, 5.5 cps, sharp transients with maximum negativity at T7 or T8 that appear either across the right temporal region or synchronously and bitemporally. *Rhythmic, midtemporal, theta discharges during drowsiness* are benign, epileptiform transients without clinical correlation. The periodic sharp waves are EKG artifact.

Discussion: Benign epileptiform transients are sharp-appearing discharges that have no clear clinical significance. Their main importance is that they can be misinterpreted as epileptogenic IEDs. In general, benign epileptiform transients fail to fulfill all criteria for IEDs. They tend to be tied to specific sleep-wake states, a susceptibility that greatly aids in recognition. Important benign epileptiform transients and their states are as follows:

Benign Epileptiform Transient	Sleep Stage
SREDA	Wake, S1
Phantom spike-wave	Wake, S1
RMTD	S1
6+14 Hz positive bursts	S1
SSS	S2

Rhythmic midtemporal theta bursts of drowsiness (RMTD), also known as rhythmic midtemporal theta discharges, are a benign epileptiform transient seen in adolescents and adults. They were originally deemed *psychomotor variant* because of the resemblance to the ictal discharges of psychomotor or temporal lobe seizures. The preferred name spells out the salient features.

Frequency. RMTD consists of bursts of rhythmic theta activity, usually 5–6 cps.

Location. Usually, RMTD shows maximum negativity at the midtemporal region. Bursts can appear synchronously and bitemporally or as asynchronous bursts that shift from side to side.

Morphology. Bursts usually have spindle-form morphology, with the largest amplitudes displayed within the middle of the burst. Individual waveforms are V-shaped. Because ongoing fast background activities are not interrupted by bursts, the summation of fast activities upon bursts often leads to a blunted or shifting morphology to the sharp end of waveforms. Unlike ictal discharges, bursts do not evolve into other frequencies or waveforms and retain their shape within and between bursts.

Activation/reactivity. RMTD is state-dependent, appearing only during initial drowsiness into stage 1 sleep. Whereas RMTD bursts are confined to this transient state, abnormal IEDs or ictal discharges often occur during other states as well.

Early investigators postulated that psychomotor variant was associated with various mental deficiencies. Currently, however, RMTD has no significant clinical correlation and is considered a normal variant of sleep.

The example also has sharp transients arising from EKG artifact. Positive identification of artifact sources aids in their distinction from true sharp discharges of cerebral origin.

Clinical Pearls

1. Benign epileptiform transients have a sharp morphology, are frequently tied to a certain sleep-wake state, and must be distinguished from IEDs.
2. RMTD are benign interictal epileptiform discharges without clinical significance.
3. Sharp transients may arise from noncerebral sources, such as EKG artifact.

REFERENCE

1. Gibbs FA, Gibbs EL: Atlas of Electroencephalography. Cambridge, MA, Addison-Wesley, 1952.

PATIENT 36

A 40-year-old epileptic man with resumption of seizures

A 40-year-old man presents with resumption of generalized tonic-clonic seizures after years of being seizure-free. Medications were phenytoin and phenobarbital.

The recording is made with the patient asleep following sleep deprivation. The sample is shown in both bipolar and referential montages.

Question: Identify the epileptiform potentials (*arrows*).

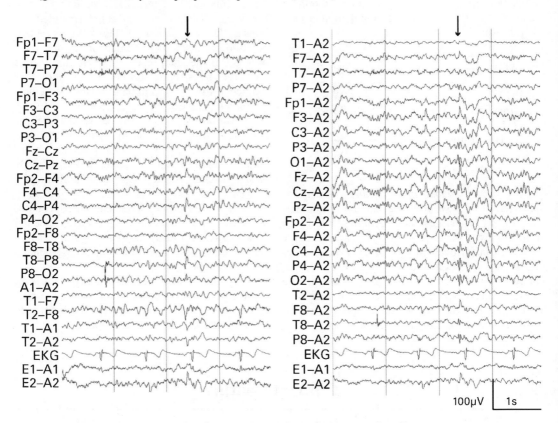

Answer: Small, sharp spikes. These are benign epileptiform transients without clinical significance.

Discussion: Small, sharp spikes (benign epileptiform transients of sleep [BETS]) are low-amplitude, biphasic, short-duration transients that occur during sleep.

Location. BETS are usually best seen in referential montages with long interelectrode distances and appear with broad potential field with maximum amplitudes across temporal regions.

Morphology. Although some waveforms feature a brief, slow afterpotential, small sharp spikes do not interrupt or distort the background. As with RMTD, small, sharp spikes usually appear unilaterally, but, given enough recording time, should appear independently on the other side.

Reactivity/state. Their appearance is confined to drowsiness and light sleep.

Clinical Pearl

Small, sharp spikes can be distinguished from IEDs by the former's short duration, biphasic morphology, and state dependence.

REFERENCE

1. Gibbs FA, Gibbs EL: Atlas of Electroencephalography. Cambridge, MA, Addison-Wesley, 1952.

PATIENT 37

A 32-year-old woman with paroxysmal paresthesia

A 32-year-old woman presents with paroxysmal paresthesia of the right face and arm. The patient has a history of migraine headaches and takes an unnamed beta-blocker antihypertensive medication for prophylaxis.

The sample is taken during the transition to drowsiness.

Question: What is the significance of the burst of sharp transients (*arrow*)?

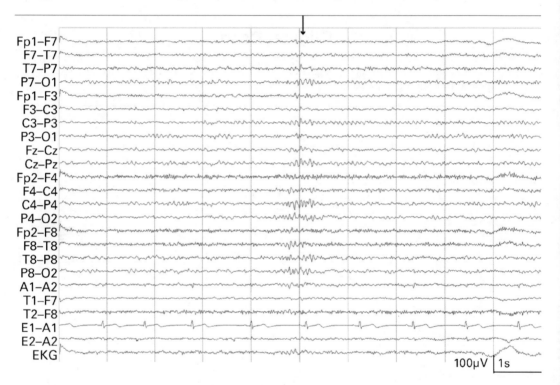

Answer: Bursts of diffusely distributed rhythmic, epileptiform theta activities, with coinciding beta activities, occur during restful wakefulness. This pattern is called *six- and fourteen-Hz positive bursts* and is a benign epileptiform transient.

Discussion: Six- and fourteen-Hz positive bursts are benign epileptiform discharges that can be mistaken for pathologic epileptiform discharges. They are most memorable for their unpronounceable synonym *ctenoid* (comb-like) waves and for a lingering but controversial association with psychiatric disease. Adolescents are the age group with the highest incidence of positive bursts.

Frequency/location. Positive bursts have a frequency around 6 cps or 14 cps, and both frequencies may appear one upon the other. They appear maximally in posterior temporal regions, with broad fields of distribution, and can appear synchronously or asynchronously.

Morphology. Brief bursts of 0.5- to 1-second duration consist of runs of sharply contoured discharges, with the sharp component having a positive polarity.

Reactivity/state. Bursts appear during restful wakefulness in its transition to drowsiness and light sleep.

Six- and fourteen-Hz positive bursts, along with small, sharp spikes and other benign epileptiform discharges, are associated with major psychiatric disease, such as schizophrenia, depression, and borderline personality disorder. Despite this association, they also occur with considerable overlap in normal individuals to the extent that they lack any helpful predictive value in diagnostic assessment. The prevailing view is that 6- and 14-Hz positive bursts and other sharp transients have no clinical import and should be designated as normal variants.

This particular example of ctenoid waves is less impressive than other published examples. One reason is that ctenoid are best seen in montages with long interelectrode distances enabling these characteristically low-amplitude discharges to better stand out from background activities. However, montages such as contralateral ear montages (left hemisphere referred to the right ear and right hemisphere referred to the left) are not generally used as often as in the past.

Clinical Pearl

6-Hz and 14-Hz positive bursts are benign epileptiform sharp transients.

REFERENCE

1. Inui K, Motomura E, Okushima R, et al: Electroencephalographic findings in patients with DSM-IV mood disorder, schizophrenia, and other psychotic disorders. Biol Psychiatry 1998; 43(1): 69–75.

PATIENT 38

A 35-year-old woman with episodic tinnitus and
loss of consciousness

A 35-year-old woman has episodes of loss of consciousness sometimes preceded by tinnitus. She is taking no medication.

The tracing is recorded with the patient awake.

Question: What is the clinical significance of the marked findings (*arrows*)?

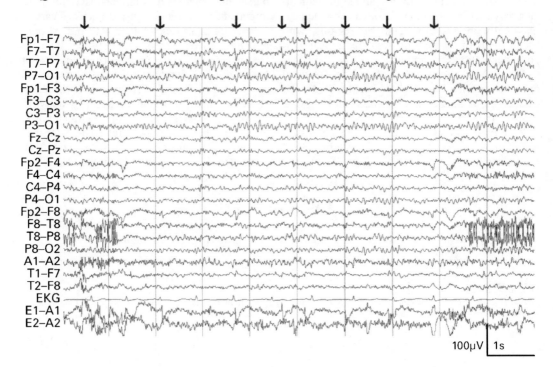

100µV | 1s

Answer: The tracing shows prominent sharp transients present at F7 that occur before lateral eye movements (confirmed by eye lead channels). These are called *lateralis muscle spicules* and are artifacts that can be mistaken for IEDs.

Discussion: As discussed before, findings that are epileptiform are not always associated with epilepsy and may not even be cerebral in origin.

One characteristic that differentiates muscle activity from cerebral activity is that muscle activity generally has a frequency >35 cps. As a consequence, transients from muscle activity are generally very sharp (35 cps = 1/35 seconds/ cycle = 29 msec/cycle). In this example, prominent, sharp transients at F7 precede apparent slow wave afterpotentials. Lateralis muscle spicules are best seen in anterior temporal leads (F7 and F8). The short duration of the transients and the characteristic slow wave artifacts confirm that the sharp and slow complexes are eye movement artifacts rather than anterior temporal sharp waves.

Clinical Pearl

Lateralis muscle spicules are short duration sharp potentials stemming from lateralis muscle artifact during lateral eye movements.

PATIENT 39

A 32-month-old boy with generalized seizures

An EEG is requested to evaluate recent onset of generalized convulsions in a 32-month-old boy with recently discovered, poorly characterized amino acid abnormalities. The patient is taking phenobarbital.

A previous EEG shows slowing of the waking alpha rhythm and persistent movement artifact from an uncooperative patient, but no IEDs are seen.

The current recording is performed after sleep deprivation, with the patient drowsy. The sample is shown in both traverse bipolar and referential montages. Supplementary electrodes at C1 and C2 are placed.

Question: Identify the transients (*arrows, a*) and their clinical significance.

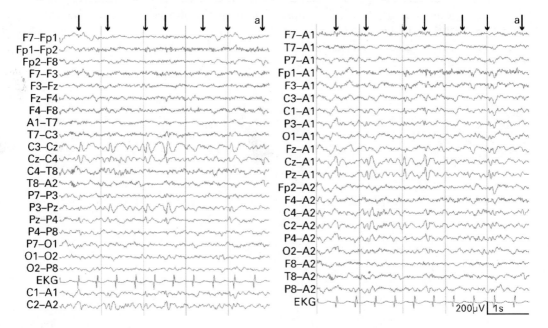

Focal Sharp Transients and Localization-Related Epilepsy

Answer: Frequent spikes are present with maximum negativity at the central vertex with potential field asymmetrically shifted to the right. One spike is located at the right central region (*a*). These are potentially epileptogenic.

Discussion: Vertex sharp transients of sleep may be difficult to distinguish from spikes that appear at the central vertex. To illustrate, seizures occur in at least 68% of children with IEDs from temporal, frontal, or occipital foci. Seizures, however, occur in only 38% of children with central IEDs. One possibility is that central spikes are less predictive of epilepsy; another is that some children may have vertex sharp transients of sleep that resemble IEDs.

Factors that distinguish vertex sharp transients of sleep from vertex spikes are:

Location. Vertex sharp transients appear synchronously and bihemispherically with maximum potential at the vertex. The potential field of vertex spikes, in contrast, is usually asymmetric. A restricted potential field is also a feature of most midline spikes, whereas most vertex sharp transients are broadly distributed.

Supplementary electrodes, C1 and C2 in this example (C1 lies 10% of the coronal distance from midline, or one-half way between Cz and C3), aid in determining a possible asymmetry in the potential field. In this case, the referential montage shows that the amplitude of the negative potential drops quickly from the vertex, but higher amplitudes are present across the right coronal midline.

Morphology. Another feature that identifies these transients as IEDs includes the classic morphology of an epileptiform negativity with a slow afterpotential, in contrast to vertex sharp transients that are broadly based and V-shaped.

Reactivity/state. Vertex sharp transients of sleep are limited to sleep, whereas central spikes may appear during various states.

Clinical Pearl

Spikes that appear at the midline must be carefully distinguished from normal vertex sharp transients of sleep. Asymmetry, restriction of field, and slow afterpotentials distinguish vertex spikes.

REFERENCE

1. Kellaway P: The incidence, significance, and natural history of spike foci in children. In Henry CE (eds): Current Clinical Neurophysiology Update on EEG and Evoked Potential. New York, Elsevier/New Holland, 1981, pp 151–175.

PATIENT 40

A 4-year-old girl with spells and cerebral palsy

An EEG is requested to help evaluate possible seizures that consist of head extension, flexion of all four extremities, and cyanosis. The 4-year-old girl has spastic cerebral palsy. The patient is taking baclofen.

The patient is asleep for much of the recording.

Question: What is the significance of the train of central transients?

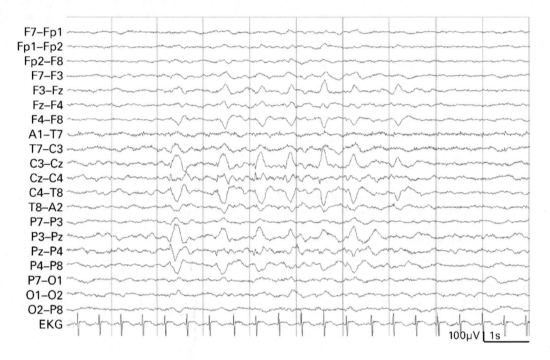

Answer: Spikes appear with maximum negativity at Cz. Several are equipotential across electrodes Cz and C4, demonstrating a shift of field to the right. Slow afterpotentials are atypical, consisting of a high-amplitude, smoothly contoured positive component and a possible negative-potential slow wave distorted by ongoing delta-theta activities. These are potentially epileptogenic—perhaps.

Discussion: Distinction among IEDs and other sharp transients is one of the main challenges of EEG interpretation. This example is particularly difficult.

Like pathologic vertex spikes, these spikes and slow waves have a potential field shifted to the right. The typical V-shape of vertex sharp transients of sleep is not present.

On the other hand, the transients lack the morphology of a typical negative potential spike and slow wave complex. Spikes are extremely brief in duration. The slow waves, in this case, are surface-negative slow potentials that follow prominent V-shaped surface positive waves.

This was the only burst of such discharges in the recording, thus comparison with more typical vertex sharp transients was not possible.

Clinical Pearls

1. The vertex sharp waves of children can be high amplitude and occur in brief trains that may be difficult to distinguish from IEDs.
2. Accurate reporting of findings and conservative interpretation allow referring physicians to draw their own conclusions in the case of ambiguous findings.

PATIENT 41

A 30-year-old woman with major depression with psychotic features

An EEG is requested to evaluate possible encephalopathy in a 30-year-old woman with major depression with psychotic features. Medications are haloperidol and mirtazapine.

The recording is made with the patient asleep.

Question: Identify the transients (*arrows*).

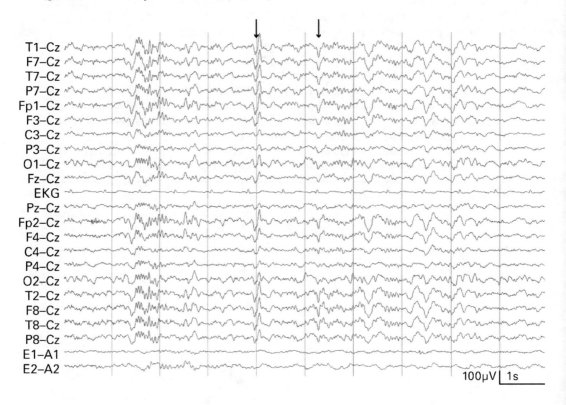

Answer: Vertex sharp transients of sleep appear widely distributed among all channels, as do sleep spindles, because of a contaminated reference.

Discussion: Montage selection is the prerogative of the EEG technologist. Selection of referential montages is particularly tricky because of possible *reference contamination*, situations in which the potential of interest has an electrical field that involves the common reference. It can lead to nonsensical phase reversals in referential montages, and, at best, distorts familiar activities into unfamiliar ones.

In the current case, selection of a Cz reference during light sleep guarantees that midline findings of sleep—vertex sharp transients, K complexes, and sleep spindles—will appear in all channels in an exaggerated fashion that falsely represents the true distribution.

Much investigation in the early days of EEG was devoted to the development of the truly uninvolved, noncerebral reference—a kind of Holy Grail. The ear electrode, the original candidate, unfortunately, is involved in many temporal potentials. In fact, many examples in this book make the use of a paired ear channel that, because of the long interelectrode distance, amplifies potentials extending from temporal regions and acts as a "signal flag" that points up or down and indicates a possible left or right IED. The paired ear channel, however, like other noncerebral sites at the nose or anterior neck, is problematic because of the amplification of EKG artifact.

The patient's state and the location of suspicious potentials are the best guides to the wise selection of reference electrodes. Left temporal abnormalities are best viewed using a reference to the right ear, and vice versa for the other side. Midline references are helpful for bitemporal abnormalities, as long as the state during which they appear is not light sleep.

With digital EEG, selection of montages can be done on the fly, so the reviewer is not locked into any one view, a distinct advantage from traditional paper-based systems.

Clinical Pearls

1. Selection of the best referential montage must take into account state and the location of abnormalities.
2. Reference electrodes should be as far away as possible from the location of the putative abnormality.

PATIENT 42

A 5-year-old girl with staring spells

A 5-year-old girl has recent onset of numerous brief spells of inattention or staring noted at school and at home. Occasionally, she has limited eye fluttering with spells, but no other automatisms are noted. Her developmental history is normal; in fact, inattention was originally ascribed to boredom in this child, who was exceeding the performance of her classmates until spells became interruptive.

The child is awake, hyperventilating, and on no medications.

Question: What is the generalized burst that interrupted hyperventilation?

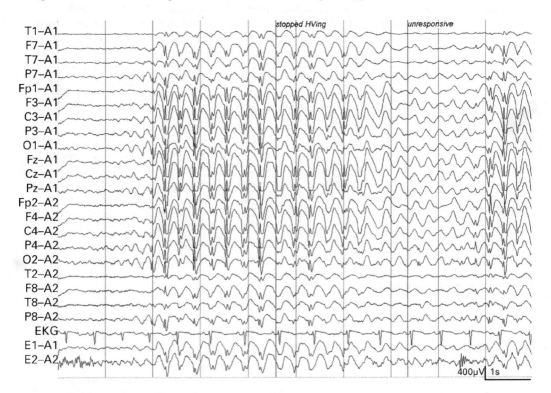

Answer: The recording shows a burst of generalized, rhythmic, high-amplitude spike-wave discharges with a frequency of 3 cps. The episode is provoked by hyperventilation, which, in turn, is interrupted by the event. Diffusely distributed, semirhythmic, medium-amplitude delta activities before the event are also present, representing hyperventilation-induced build-up. This tracing is diagnostic for a generalized, typical absence seizure and is most consistent with *childhood absence epilepsy* (CAE).

Discussion: CAE (petit mal, pyknolepsy) is an idiopathic generalized epilepsy marked by absence seizures. Age of onset ranges from 4–8 years, with a peak at 5–6 years, corresponding to kindergarten in the United States.

Patients with CAE experience *absence seizures*, episodes of behavioral arrest, unresponsiveness, and staring that are sometimes perceived as inattention or daydreaming. Because the seizures are typically brief (less than 15 seconds in about 75% of patients), a history of the spells' resolution with intervention—"shaking them out of a spell"—is often unreliable. Mild automatisms, such as eyelid fluttering or blinking, limited orofacial automatisms, or mild alterations in extensor tone, can be present.

Absence seizures may occur at a daily frequency too numerous to count, a historical point that is helpful in their distinction from complex partial seizures that occur at a much less frequent rate. Patients usually have no clear antecedent CNS injuries and usually have normal, even supernormal, cognitive abilities. Clinical exam is normal, but hyperventilation can provoke absence seizures in more than half of patients with CAE, a helpful office technique. More than 75% of patients with CAE enjoy total remission of seizures by age 14. Poor prognostic factors for seizure remission include cognitive impairment, susceptibility to hyperventilation, myoclonus with absence, and later age of onset. Patients with continuing absence seizures usually develop generalized tonic-clonic seizures or myoclonic seizures.

The EEG is often diagnostic in CAE.

Frequency/amplitude. The characteristic finding is rhythmic, *3 cps spike-wave* bursts. Amplitudes range from 300–600 μV.

Location. Bursts are generalized, synchronous, and symmetric, usually with anterior dominance in amplitude.

Morphology. Rhythmic spike-slow wave complexes, the classic "dart and dome," are difficult to mistake for other patterns. Longer runs usually demonstrate that frequency, amplitude, and morphology evolve. Initially, the rate of spike-waves ranges between 3 and 3.5 cps, and spikes may attain higher voltages than the following wave. Initial amplitudes are at their highest. At the end of bursts, frequencies may drop to 2.5–3 cps, spikes may fade in amplitude or even disappear, and waves may drop slightly in amplitude. No postictal slowing is present.

Activation. Hyperventilation induces spike-wave bursts in about 80% of patients with CAE. One characteristic of 3 cps spike-wave is that bursts during non-REM sleep usually become shorter, less regular, and can feature multiple spikes. Viewing discharges only during sleep may lead to a misdiagnosis of atypical spike-wave discharges. Findings that may be confused with 3 cps spike-wave, hypersynchrony of sleep, atypical spike-wave discharges, rhythmic delta activity, and fast multispike-wave discharges will be discussed in separate sections.

Obvious clinical changes, such as behavioral arrest seen in the interruption of hyperventilation described previously, may not be present. Confirmation of transient impairment may require response testing.

Occipital intermittent rhythmic delta activity (OIRDA) is a frequent finding as well in patients with CAE.

Clinical Pearls

1. Typical 3 cps spike-wave bursts are the key EEG finding in CAE.
2. CAE, when defined by typical spike-wave discharges and not present with cognitive impairment or myoclonus, resolves without residual effects in the majority of children.

REFERENCES

1. Sato S, Dreifuss FE, J Kirby DD, Palesch Y: Long-term follow-up of absence seizures. Neurology 1983; 33:1590–1595.
2. Weir B: The morphology of the spike-wave complex. Electroencephalography Clin Neurophysiol 1965; 19:284–290.
3. Wirrel E, Camfield C, Camfield P, et al: Long-term prognosis of typical childhood absence epilepsy: remission or progression to juvenile myoclinic epilepsy. Neurology 1996; 47:912–918.

PATIENT 43

A 7-year-old girl with staring spells

A 7-year-old girl presents with 2–4 staring spells a day. She is performing poorly in school this year after having been successful during the previous year. She takes no medications.
The recording is performed during hyperventilation.

Question: What is the finding accompanying this spell of inattention? The excerpt shows the middle 5 seconds from parasaggital channels (*bar*).

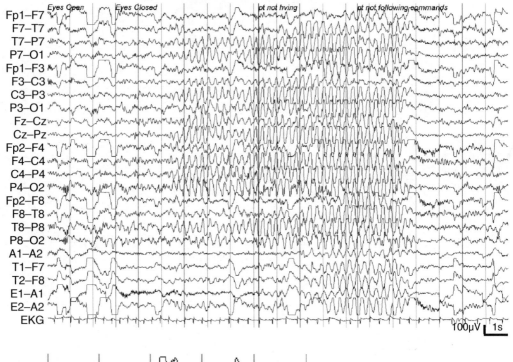

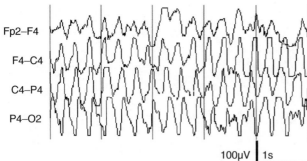

Answer: Profound hyperventilation-induced build-up is interrupted by transient inattention. Hyperventilation-induced inattention and rhythmic delta activity (delta absence) probably represents a normal, physiologic response to hypocapnia in individuals who are not suspected of having absence epilepsy.

Discussion: Delta absence is a term coined to describe patients undergoing evaluation for staring spells who have episodes of high-amplitude, rhythmic delta activity induced during hyperventilation. Response testing demonstrates that subjects have impaired consciousness during what has since been dubbed *hyperventilation-induced high-amplitude rhythmic slowing* (HIHARS); in other words, build-up. In the original report, anticonvulsant medications successfully treated staring spells, raising the possibility that rhythmic delta activity was a form of an ictal discharge.

Subsequent investigators, however, duplicated both impairment of consciousness and HIHARS in nonepileptic children, suggesting that HIHARS and accompanying inattention is a nonepileptic, physiologic response to hypocapnia.

Later work showed that clinical symptoms differ in those patients whose absence seizures with 3 cps spike-wave were activated by hyperventilation and those whose inattention were marked by HIHARS. Those with 3 cps bursts were more likely to have automatisms during bursts, whereas those with HIHARS merely yawned or fidgeted.

In this light, HIHARS most likely represents a nonepileptic phenomenon in subjects who are not suspected of having absence seizures. In these patients, HIHARS is a variant of normal hyperventilation-induced build-up. On the other hand, those with possible absence seizures and HIHARS should be investigated further to uncover further evidence of absence seizures, such as another attempt at recording characteristic 3 cps spike-wave bursts.

Hyperventilation-induced buildup may be distinguished from 3 cps spike-wave bursts by the former's lack of spikes. As seen in the excerpt, ongoing past activities occasionally persist through bursts of delta activity, giving the false appearance of spikes that do not maintain a clear, consistent timing relationship with the slow waves.

Clinical Pearl

HIHARS is a variant of normal hyperventilation-induced build-up in patients not suspected of absence seizures.

REFERENCES

1. Epstein MA, Duchowny M, Jayakar P, et al: Altered responsiveness during hyperventilation-induced EEG slowing: A nonepileptic phenomenon in normal children. Epilepsia 1994; 35(6):1204–1207.
2. Lee SI, Kirby D: Absence seizure with generalized rhythmic delta activity. Epilepsia 1988; 29(3):262–267.
3. Lum LM, Connolly MB, Wong PK: Hyperventilation-induced high-amplitude rhythmic slowing with altered awareness: A video-EEG comparison with absence seizures. Epilepsia 2002; 43:1372–1378.

PATIENT 44

A 41-year-old woman with tonic-clonic convulsions after motor vehicle accident

An EEG is requested to evaluate spells that resemble tonic-clonic convulsions in a 41-year-old woman the day after a motor vehicle accident. She is apparently unharmed but presents with recurrent spells and unresponsiveness in the emergency room where she receives intravenous midazolam.

The recording is performed several hours after midazolam administration, with the patient awake. The sample is shown in both bipolar and referential montages.

Question: What is the significance of sharp transients noted under the bars?

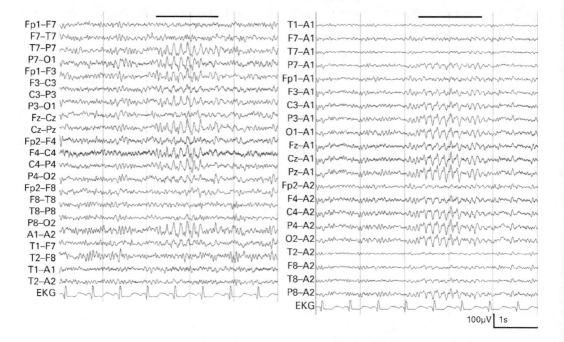

100µV 1s

Answer: Bursts of diffusely distributed rhythmic theta activities occur during restful wakefulness. Small spikes occur in relationship to theta frequency "slow waves." This pattern is called *phantom spike-wave* and is a benign epileptiform transient.

Discussion: Phantom spike-waves (6-Hz spike-waves) are benign epileptiform discharges that can be mistaken for pathologic spike-wave discharges.

Frequency/location. They appear in bursts with a frequency around 6 cps. Bursts are brief, only lasting 1–2 seconds and appear diffusely across the scalp with varying predominant locations among individuals.

Morphology. The *phantom spike* refers to the small spike associated with the theta activity "slow wave" that often comes and goes during bursts.

Reactivity. Phantom spike-wave occurs during restful wakefulness and initial drowsiness. They disappear with light sleep.

The main points of distinction between phantom spike-waves and IEDs are that phantom spike-waves fail to evolve temporally or spatially and are obligately linked to specific states of restful wakefulness or the transition to light sleep.

Although older literature suggests that phantom spike-wave is a possible indicator of neurologic or social pathology, phantom spike-wave has no significant clinical correlate and is considered a benign epileptiform transient.

In this case, the patient was admitted to an inpatient EEG monitoring unit; continuous video-EEG captured several spells that were not accompanied by ictal discharges. In the situation in which spells are acute and frequent, prompt continuous video-EEG may stave off unnecessary treatment with anticonvulsant medications.

Clinical Pearl

Phantom spike-wave is a benign finding of diffusely distributed bursts of theta activities, sometimes occurring with small spike discharges.

PATIENT 45

A 29-year-old man with medically intractable generalized seizures

A 29-year-old man has a 10-year history of seizures consisting of abrupt loss of consciousness and staring, followed by brief, bilateral tonic posturing of the upper extremities. Frequent, generalized tonic-clonic seizures follow initial symptoms. Most seizures occur nocturnally in clusters. Current medications are lamotrigine and topiramate.

The recording is made with the patient asleep.

Question: Does the finding here of diffuse spike-wave discharges support a diagnosis of generalized epilepsy?

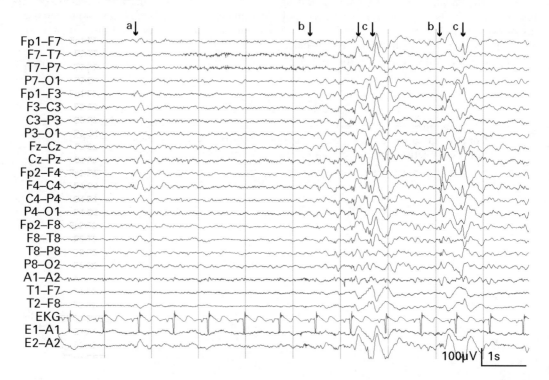

Generalized Discharges and Generalized Epilepsy

Answer: Focal spikes and slowing at F4 (*arrow a*) before the spike-wave burst, along with initial slow waves or spikes at F4 (*arrows b*) that precede the burst of diffusely distributed spike-wave complexes (*arrows c*) suggest a focal epileptic lesion that spreads rapidly and bilaterally.

Discussion: *Secondary bilateral synchrony* designates an EEG finding of generalized and synchronous epileptiform discharges that arise not from generalized epilepsy but from a focal epileptic lesion.

Secondary bilateral synchrony should be suspected when generalized spike-wave discharges occur in special relationship to focal findings. Focal IEDs distinct in morphology and recurrent in location are present in addition to generalized discharges. Focal IEDs precede and evolve into secondarily generalized discharges. Generalized spike-wave bursts in secondary bilateral synchrony usually occur in frequencies slower than typical 3 cps spike-wave bursts.

Such foci are usually located in the frontal lobes. Frontal lobe seizures may occur briefly and frequently without aura, may be accompanied by subtle asymmetric motor posturing, and may not be followed by postictal confusion. On the other hand, other frontal lobe seizures present with complex, bizarre motor automatisms or focal clonic motor activity. Frontal lobe seizures also tend to occur during sleep and to secondarily generalize.

Difficulties arise in the diagnosis between frontal lobe epilepsy with secondary bilateral synchrony and primary generalized epilepsy because both may show interictal focal findings on EEG. In the case of idiopathic generalized epilepsies, about 20% of patients with *juvenile myoclonic epilepsy* demonstrate focal spikes. More severe generalized epilepsies can demonstrate focal abnormalities; patients with *Lennox-Gastaut syndrome* may have complex partial seizures and can demonstrate interictal focal slowing.

Several techniques may help in differentiating focal from generalized epilepsies following EEGs that demonstrate possible secondary bilateral synchrony. In patients with generalized or multifocal epilepsies, focal findings tend to be evanescent and usually do not appear on repeat recordings. Examination of generalized bursts of suspected focal origin can be viewed with increased paper speed in an attempt to determine close timing of any initial activity. Bipolar montages may be helpful in minimizing synchronous activity and drawing the eye to focal findings. Ultimately, continuous video-EEG recordings that capture the events in question may be necessary to distinguish between primary and secondary generalized seizures.

The assignment of intractable epilepsy patients to either primary generalized or localization-related epilepsies aids in guiding therapy. Certain anticonvulsants, carbamazepine and tiagabine, in particular, may exacerbate seizures or provoke status epilepticus in susceptible patients with primary generalized epilepsies. Patients with localization-related epilepsies, even with findings of rapid secondary generalization, may benefit from consideration of epilepsy surgery.

Clinical Pearls

1. Secondary bilateral synchrony designates an EEG finding of bilateral and synchronous epileptiform discharges that arise from a focal epileptic lesion and rapidly generalize.

2. Criteria for secondary bilateral synchrony include that focal IEDs appear temporally and morphologically separate from generalized discharges, and immediately precede generalized discharges.

REFERENCES

1. Murthy JM, Rao CM, Meena AK: Clinical observations of juvenile myoclonic epilepsy in 131 patients: A study in South India. Seizure 1998; 7(1):43–47.
2. Perucca E, Gram L, Avanzini G, Dulac O: Antiepileptic drugs as a cause of worsening seizures. Epilepsia 1998; 39:5–17.

PATIENT 46

A 12-year-old girl with light-provoked seizures and morning myoclonic seizures

A 12-year-old girl has a generalized tonic-clonic seizure while watching cartoons on TV the morning after a late bedtime and sleepover at a friend's house. She notes habitual and frequent jerks of the upper extremities, clustered in the morning during breakfast and her morning shower. Her mother also has morning myoclonus.

The EEG was recorded with the patient awake. Photic stimulation, a rapidly flashing strobe light, is designated in the "photic" channel.

Question: What are the findings and the epileptic syndrome that is most likely associated with it?

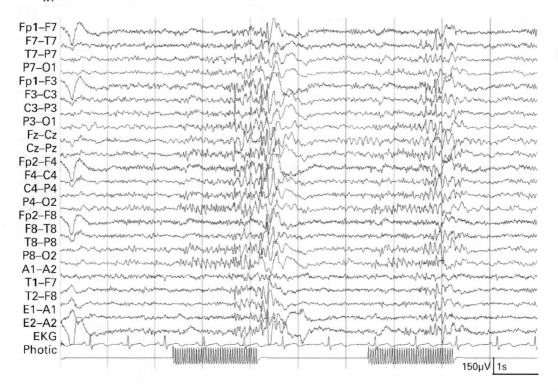

Answer: The recording shows a burst of generalized, polyspike wave discharges occurring during and outlasting photic stimulation, defining a photoparoxysmal response. The clinical and electrographic findings are consistent with *juvenile myoclonic epilepsy (JME)*.

Discussion: JME (epilepsy of Janz) is an idiopathic, generalized epilepsy marked by myoclonic seizures. Age of onset ranges from 12–19 years, with peak onset between 15 and 16 years. Intelligence is normal. Family history is strongly positive. Family members may experience only minor symptoms, such as morning myoclonus, often identified as "normal" to those who have no reason to think otherwise.

Patients with JME experience various generalized seizures: myoclonic seizures (typically clustered in the morning near awakening), generalized tonic clonic seizures, and absence seizures. Seizures in JME are often susceptible to flashing lights or sleep deprivation. JME responds readily to treatment and is associated with excellent cognitive and functional outcome. Remission is rare. Most patients require lifelong treatment.

Generalized *polyspike-wave* discharges (fast spike-wave, multiple spike-wave) are the typical IEDs seen in JME. Sometimes distinguishing interictal from ictal discharges is difficult, because accompanying jerks may be subtle in some patients.

Frequency/location. The generalized, often anteriorly dominant, bursts of polyspike-wave discharges typically occur at a much faster rate than typical spike-wave seizures in CAE. Spikes occur in ~5 cps or faster within bursts, tending to slow within single bursts.

Morphology. As shown in the excerpt, the morphology of individual discharges can vary within the same run. Bursts of spike-wave discharges can appear intermixed with bursts of spikes, typically in rhythmic runs in the alpha or theta range, followed by prominent negative-potential slow waves.

Activation. As demonstrated in the present case, photic stimulation provokes a burst of generalized, polyspike-wave discharges—*photoparoxysmal responses*—that outlast photic stimuli. Note that the technologist has terminated each block of stimuli prematurely (usually blocks are 10 seconds long in our laboratory) for fear of provoking generalized tonic-clonic seizures. Because treatment with anticonvulsant medications can decrease the incidence of abnormal discharges in the case of idiopathic generalized epilepsies, reasonable attempts at a confirmatory EEG before treatment is recommended. Finally, because seizures in JME are more likely to occur in the morning or after awakening, scheduling recordings in the morning after sleep deprivation may further improve sensitivity.

Photosensitivity provokes photoparoxysmal responses in about 50% of women with JME and in about 25% of men. Positive responses are much higher in those who do not experience generalized convulsions (100% women, 50% men).

JME must be differentiated from progressive myoclonic epilepsies, an assortment of diseases associated with neurologic deterioration, myoclonus epilepsy, and poor outcome. As opposed to many of these diseases, the background EEG in JME is normal.

Clinical Pearls

1. Juvenile myoclonic epilepsy is a syndrome of adolescent onset of generalized seizures, usually myoclonic and generalized tonic clonic, associated with excellent response to treatment, cognitive sparing, and lack of remission.

2. The IED seen in JME is the generalized polyspike-wave discharge. The finding occurs spontaneously and during photic stimulation. Polyspike-wave discharges during photic stimulation are called photoparoxysmal responses.

REFERENCES

1. Janz D: The idiopathic generalized epilepsies of adolescence with childhood and juvenile age of onset. Epilepsia 1997; 38:4–11.
2. Janz D, Durner M, Beck-Mannagetta G, Pantazis G: Family studies on the genetics of juvenile myoclonic epilepsy (epilepsy with impulsive petit mal). In Beck-Mannagetta G, Anderson VE, Doose H, Janz D (eds): Genetics of the Epilepsies. Berlin, Springer, 1989, pp 43–52.
3. Wolf P, Gooses R: Relation of photosensitive epilepsy to epileptic syndromes. J Neurol Neurosurg Psychiatry 1986; 49:1386–1391.

PATIENT 47

A 14-year-old girl with photic discomfort

A 14-year-old girl has visual discomfort provoked by working on computers. Family history is significant for epilepsy in an older sister with JME.

The recording is performed with the patient awake and on no medications.

Question: What does the response during photic stimulation indicate?

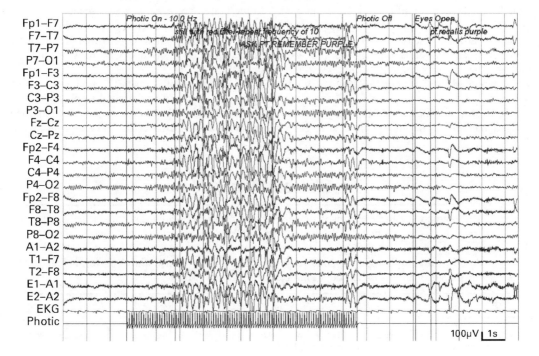

Answer: The burst of generalized polyspike-wave discharges does not outlast photic stimulation. Self-limited photoparoxysmal responses have unclear clinical significance.

Discussion: The most significant abnormal response during photic stimulation is the photoparoxysmal response, a burst of generalized polyspike-wave discharges provoked by photic stimulation.

Photoparoxysmal responses are traditionally divided into two groups, those that continue after photic stimulation ends ("prolonged"), and those that cease after photic stimulation ("self-limited"). Prolonged photoparoxysmal responses are thought to have a significant association with idiopathic generalized epilepsy. JME has the highest incidence of association with photoparoxysmal responses. It is one of the few EEG findings that are not equally split between the sexes; women have a higher incidence of photosensitivity.

In contrast, self-limited photoparoxysmal responses may occur in nonepileptic subjects or asymptomatic family members. No data suggest just how "prolonged" is significant. Many recommend that one waveform, that is, one full polyspike-wave, after cessation of stimulation is abnormally prolonged. Other studies show a significant association between photoparoxysmal responses and idiopathic, generalized epilepsies regardless of the self-limited or prolonged nature of the discharge.

A conservative approach is to interpret self-limited photoparoxysmal responses as those with unclear clinical significance, noting that familial traits may allow their expression. The finding must be placed in context with the symptoms of the patient.

In this particular patient, photoparoxysmal responses remained self-limited to photic blocks. No spontaneous IEDs were observed. Symptoms gradually attenuated over the next year in follow-up.

Clinical Pearls

1. Photoparoxysmal responses of generalized polyspike-wave discharges that last beyond blocks of photic stimuli are seen in JME and in other idiopathic, generalized epilepsies.

2. Self-limited photoparoxysmal responses that do not outlast stimuli have unclear clinical significance and can be an indicator of a familial trait.

REFERENCES

1. Puglia J, Brenner R, Soso M: Relationship between prolonged and self-limited photoparoxysmal responses and seizure incidence: Study and review. J Clin Neurophysiol 1992; 9(1):137–144.
2. Reilly EW, Peters JF: Relationship of some varieties of electroencephalographic photosensitivity to clinical convulsive disorders. Neurology 1977; 23:1045–1057.
3. Wolf P, Gooses R: Relation of photosensitive epilepsy to epileptic syndromes. J Neurol Neurosurg Psychiatry 1986; 49:1386–1391.

PATIENT 48

A 12-week-old female infant with spells of bilateral limb
extension and trunk flexion

A 12-week-old female infant is delivered at term via an uncomplicated pregnancy. She develops spells of bilateral limb extension and trunk flexion after first having spells of rightward head deviation and right arm extension. Coinciding with spells is the mother's report of decreased activity and feeding. The patient takes no medications.

The recording is made with the patient awake and asleep. Clinical sleep is shown in the 20-second sample.

Question: What is the epileptic syndrome?

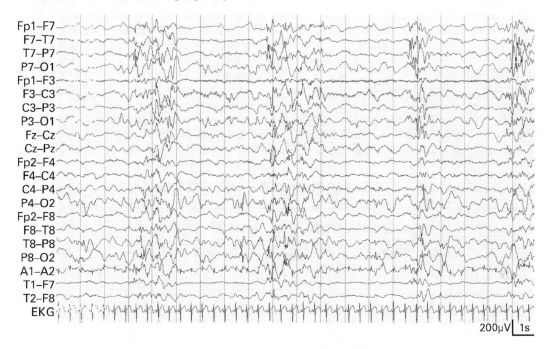

Answer: The EEG shows no age-appropriate activities of sleep; instead, recurrent high-amplitude bursts of activity are interrupted by periods of relatively suppressed activity. Suppression-burst with episodes of infantile spasms are consistent with Ohtahara syndrome.

Discussion: Epileptic encephalopathy defines a syndrome of decline in function or regression in development, epileptic seizures, and stereotypic patterns of interictal activity on EEG. Characteristics of each element of this triad depend on age and may evolve from one to another. Epileptic encephalopathies should be considered as age-specific pathologic responses to various brain injuries. Epileptic encephalopathies can be classified as idiopathic, symptomatic, or cryptogenic epilepsies, depending upon the specific etiology.

Ohtahara syndrome, also known as *early infantile epileptic encephalopathy* (EIEE), occurs within the first 3 months of life and is marked by developmental regression, infantile spasms or partial seizures, and a suppression-burst pattern on the interictal EEG.

Ohtahara syndrome should be distinguished from *early neonatal myoclonic encephalopathy* (ENME). Both syndromes appear in the neonatal period, and both are marked by suppression-burst. ENME presents with massive myoclonus, rather than infantile spasms. ENME is usually caused by progressive and often devastating etiologies stemming from inborn errors of metabolism. Glycine encephalopathy is a classic cause of ENME presenting with suppression-burst on EEG.

Ohtahara syndrome, on the other hand, is often caused by cerebral dysgenesis and can have idiopathic causes, implying a better outcome. Response to treatment (ACTH in the United States, often vigabatrin outside the United States) is also more variable than in ENME. Progression to later epileptic encephalopathies is common. Follow-up EEGs are helpful in determining the course of therapy, and resolution of suppression-burst early in the course is thought to be a good prognostic sign.

This patient was treated with ACTH injections. Infantile spasms resolved, but by age 6 months the child was not progressing developmentally. No specific etiology was uncovered.

Clinical Pearls

1. Epileptic encephalopathies are syndromes defined by the triad of clinical regression, seizure type, and interictal EEG pattern.
2. Ohtahara syndrome is diagnosed by neonatal regression, infantile spasms, and suppression-burst pattern on interictal EEG.

REFERENCES

1. Tharp BR: Neonatal seizures and syndromes. Epilepsia 2002; 43:S2–S10.
2. Yamatogi Y, Ohtahara S: Early-infantile epileptic encephalopathy with suppression-bursts: Ohtahara syndrome; its overview referring to our 16 cases. Brain Dev 2002; 24:13–23.

PATIENT 49

An 8-month-old male infant with congenital abnormalities and spells of bilateral limb flexion

An 8-month-old male infant has midline congenital abnormalities and presents with developmental delay and spells of bilateral limb and trunk flexion that cluster upon awakening from naps. The patient is taking no medications.

The recording is made with the patient awake after having awoken from a nap. An episode of trunk and bilateral limb flexion ("body jerk") is noted by the technologist.

Question: What are the EEG findings and the epileptic syndrome?

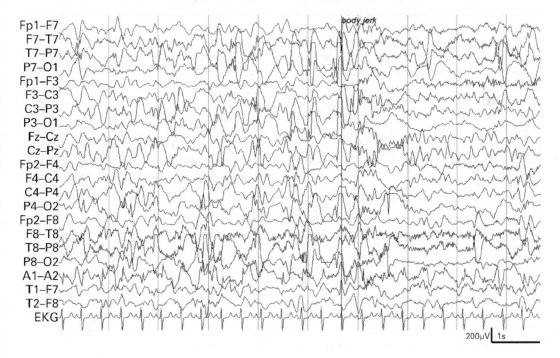

Answer: Hypsarrhythmia. Attenuation that corresponds to an infantile spasm is an *electro-decremental seizure.* These findings are consistent with West syndrome.

Discussion: The triad of developmental delay, hypsarrhythmia, and infantile spasms defines *West syndrome.* West syndrome is an epileptic encephalopathy that affects infants and young children from ages 3 months to 2 years, with peak onset at ages 8–9 months. *Infantile spasms* consist of abrupt and brief flexion of the upper limbs and trunk, sometimes along with the legs. The rapid flexions lead to the obsolete terms "clasp-knife" or "salaam" seizures. Occasionally, infantile spasms occur as extensor events. Seizures often cluster at transitions from sleep to wakefulness.

As in Ohtahara syndrome, various etiologies are associated with West syndrome, although many are eventually classified as cryptogenic. Tuberous sclerosis is an important cause of symptomatic West syndrome. Although EEG changes are diffuse, functional neuroimaging may reveal a lesion amenable to epilepsy surgery. Outcome in West syndrome is determined by the underlying cause, although control of the seizures and hypsarrhythmia—usually with ACTH in the United States and with vigabatrin elsewhere—is associated with better cognitive outcome. About a third of patients progress to the next epileptic encephalopathy, Lennox-Gastaut syndrome.

Hypsarrhythmia means "mountainous activities." Normal background activities are absent; instead, continuous arrhythmic, high-amplitude, asynchronous delta activities with independent, multifocal spike discharges are present. Many interpreters specify a minimum amplitude of 200 μV to qualify as hypsarrhythmia. Sleep may cause continuous hypsarrhythmia to fragment, allowing periods of lower-amplitude semirhythmic delta and theta activities to emerge. When delta and theta background activities are present during both sleep and wakefulness, interspersed between runs of hypsarrhythmia, the pattern is traditionally called *modified hypsarrhythmia.* Despite the apparent "improvement" by the emergence of background activity, modified hypsarrhythmia has the same clinical import as continuous hypsarrhythmia.

An abrupt attenuation that follows a high-amplitude sharp-and-slow wave complex, electrodecremental seizure, is the usual marker of an infantile spasm.

This patient was eventually found to have multiple heterotopias, polymicrogyria, and dysmyelination on neuroimaging. ACTH injections resolved hypsarrhythmia and spasms, but the child did not survive because of complications due to other malformations.

Clinical Pearls

1. West syndrome is a triad of infantile developmental regression or delay, infantile spasms, and hypsarrhythmia.
2. Hypsarrhythmia is defined as continuous, high-amplitude, arrhythmic, asynchronous delta activities with interspersed independent, multiple spikes.

REFERENCES

1. Asano E, Chugani DC, Juhasz C, Muzik O: Surgical treatment of West syndrome. Brain Dev 2001; 23:668–676.
2. Dulac O: Epileptic encephalopathy. Epilepsia 2001; 43:S23–S26.
3. Gibbs FA, Gibbs EL: Atlas of Electroencephalography. Cambridge, MA, Addison-Wesley, 1952.

PATIENT 50

A 3-year-old girl with developmental delay and "drop attacks"

A 3-year-old girl with developmental delay is referred for evaluation of recent onset of drop attacks, abrupt loss of tone causing her to fall forward. She is taking valproate.

The recording is made with the patient awake. The G2 input is the averaged ear reference (A1 + A2).

Question: What are the EEG findings and the epileptic syndrome?

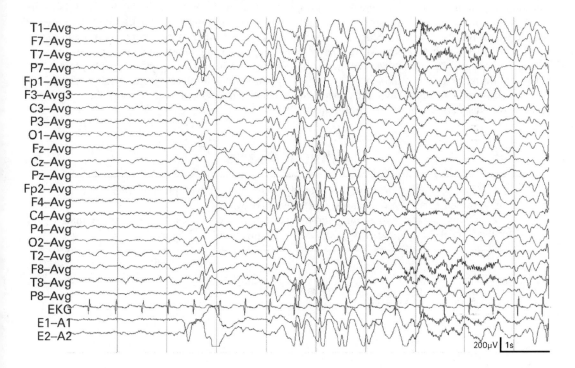

Answer: Slow spike-wave consistent with Lennox-Gastaut syndrome.

Discussion: The triad of developmental delay, astatic seizures, and atypical spike-wave bursts defines *Lennox-Gastaut syndrome* (LGS). LGS is an epileptic encephalopathy that affects children from ages 2–18. As in other epileptic encephalopathies, LGS can result from idiopathic, symptomatic, or cryptogenic causes. Many patients with LGS had a previous epileptic encephalopathy, such as West syndrome.

Authorities emphasize different seizures in Lennox-Gastaut. *Astatic seizures* (drop attacks) certainly can be the most difficult to treat and the most injurious. Atypical absences, featuring more myoclonus and automatisms than typical absence seizures, frequently occur, as well as tonic and tonic-clonic seizures. Most now refer to the various mixed, generalized seizures that often remain refractory to treatment.

Slow spike-wave, bursts of rhythmic generalized spike-wave discharges, must be differentiated from typical 3 cps spike-wave bursts. Slow spike-wave bursts have a frequency of 2–2.5 cps, as opposed to 3–3.5 cps of typical spike-wave. Often the "spikes" of slow spike-wave bursts are broader than 70 milliseconds. Bursts of slow spike-wave may be also less rhythmically regular than typical spike-wave. Slow spike-wave bursts in LGS have no clinical accompaniment, whereas typical spike-wave bursts usually denote clinical and electrographic seizures. These differences lead to the syndrome's original name of *petit mal variant*.

Other abnormalities in the EEG of LGS include abnormally slow background activities of wakefulness and independent, multifocal spikes. Sleep recordings may contain bursts of low-amplitude, generalized, rhythmic alpha-beta activities, similar to electrodecremental seizures, that usually mark occurrence of tonic seizures.

Clinical Pearls

1. Lennox-Gastaut syndrome is a triad of childhood developmental regression or delay, mixed generalized seizures, and slow spike-wave.

2. A slow spike-wave is an interictal pattern in Lennox-Gastaut syndrome that, unlike typical 3 cps spike-wave, occurs at a frequency of 2–2.5 cps.

REFERENCES

1. Dulac O: Epileptic encephalopathy. Epilepsia 2001; 43:S23–S26.
2. Gibbs FA, Gibbs EL: Atlas of Electroencephalography. Cambridge, MA, Addison-Wesley, 1952.

PATIENT 51

A 4-year-old boy with progressive neurologic deterioration and myoclonic epilepsy

Ongoing seizure activity is questioned in a 4-year-old boy with the subacute onset of myoclonic seizures and cognitive deterioration. He is admitted for nearly continuous generalized and migratory myoclonic seizures. Chronic anticonvulsants include lamotrigine and zonisamide after the patient failed trials of valproate and topiramate.

The recording is performed with the patient awake but unable to follow commands. He is given intravenous lorazepam 3 hours before the recording.

Questions: What is the finding? With what epilepsy syndrome is it associated?

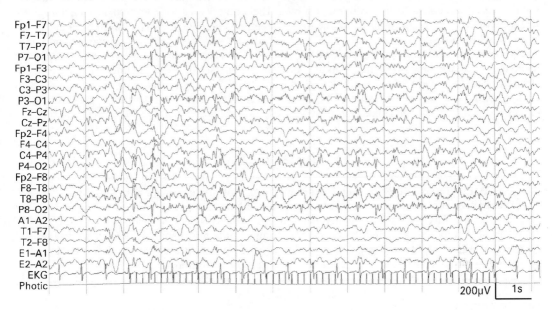

Answers: The finding is occipital spikes evoked by photic stimulation (high-amplitude photic driving responses). Giant visual evoked potentials and somatosensory evoked potentials may be seen in certain progressive myoclonus epilepsies.

Discussion: Progressive myoclonus epilepsies (PME) encompass a group of symptomatic, generalized epilepsies denoted by cognitive deterioration to the point of dementia, neurologic deficits referable to multiple systems, and myoclonic seizures. Myoclonic seizures can be massive, generalized jerking, or migratory, segmental myoclonus. Partial seizures, especially from the occipital lobe, are also prevalent.

Diseases causing PME include Unverricht-Lundborg disease (Baltic myoclonus), sialidosis (cherry-red spot myoclonus), Gaucher's disease (glucocerebroside beta-glucosidase deficiency), mitochondrial encephalopathy with ragged red fibers (MERRF), Lafora's disease, and neuronal ceroid lipofuscinosis.

The background EEG in patients with PME is marked by replacement of normal waking and sleeping activities with abnormally slow and disorganized theta and delta activities. Multifocal or generalized spikes, polyspikes, and atypical spike-wave discharges are often present. Occipital spikes can be present.

Although most patients with PME have unremarkable evoked potentials, some patients, especially those with neuronal ceroid lipofuscinosis, have abnormally high amplitude evoked potentials. High-amplitude somatosensory evoked potentials, so-called giant SSEPs, are thought to reflect a state of heightened cortical excitability. Analogous to giant SSEPs, high-amplitude pattern reversal visual evoked potentials can also be present.

In this case, the patient has the late infantile subtype of neuronal ceroid lipofuscinosis (Jansky-Bielschowsky disease). Prominent occipital spikes, reminiscent of giant visual-evoked potentials, were recorded only during slow-frequency photic stimulation. Whereas photoparoxysmal response are most typically evoked at stimulation frequencies of 10–20 Hz, high-amplitude driving responses in susceptible individuals with PME are best seen at slower driving frequencies between 2 and 5 Hz.

Clinical Pearls

1. Progressive myoclonic epilepsies are a group of diseases marked by progressive cognitive and neurologic deterioration and myoclonic epilepsy.

2. The EEG in PME is distinguished by abnormally slow and disorganized background activities, and multifocal spike, polyspike, or atypical spike-wave discharges.

3. High-amplitude ("giant") posterior driving responses evoked at slow photic driving frequencies can be seen in neuronal ceroid lipofuscinosis.

REFERENCES

1. Pampiglione G, Harden A: So-called neuronal ceroid lipofuscinosis: Neurophysiological studies in 60 children. J Neurol Neurosurg Psychiatry 1977; 40:323–330.
2. Scaioli V, Nardocci N: A pathophysiological study of neuronal ceroid lipofuscinoses in 17 patients: Critical review and methodological proposal. Neurol Sci 2000; 21:S89–S92.
3. Schmitt B, Thun-Hohenstein L, Molinari L, et al: Somatosensory evoked potentials with high cortical amplitudes: Clinical data in 31 children. Neuropediatrics 1994; 25:74–84.

PATIENT 52

A 7-month-old girl with generalized seizures after anoxic encephalopathy

A 7-month-old girl status post anoxic encephalopathy developed generalized tonic clonic and myoclonic seizures. Medications are phenobarbital and levetiracetam.

In an attempt to catch a seizure, a prolonged recording—2 hours total—was performed in the laboratory.

Question: What are the locations of spikes labeled at time *a*, *b*, and *c*?

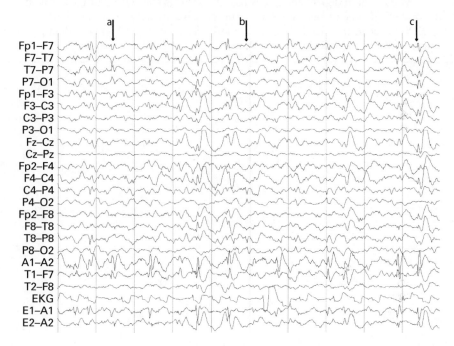

Answer: *(a)* Left midtemporal, *(b)* right parietal, and *(c)* bifrontal regions.

Discussion: IEDs that occur in several different locations with no clear relationship to each other are termed *multifocal, independent spikes*.

Like the patient shown here, multifocal independent spikes usually occur in subjects with static or progressive encephalopathies. Most patients have frequent seizures that are medically intractable, and most are mentally retarded. Because of this association with severe seizures, some EEGers designate multifocal, independent spikes as "highly epileptogenic."

In this patient with anoxic encephalopathy, background EEG activities of diffuse, unreactive arrhythmic delta activities reflect the severe involvement of the disease's effect on white matter.

Clinical Pearls

1. Multifocal, independent spikes usually occur in the setting of background slowing of the EEG in patients with static or progressive diffuse or multifocal brain disease.

2. Multifocal, independent spikes are usually considered highly epileptogenic because of their strong association with medically–intractable epileptic seizures.

PATIENT 53

A 28-year-old woman after a single seizure

A 28-year-old previously healthy woman presents after a single event of staring and confusion with mild oral-facial automatisms after an all-night party. She has no epilepsy risk factors, such as febrile convulsions, head trauma, or CNS infection. Family history is unremarkable for epilepsy. Neurologic examination is normal. A previous EEG is normal. She is taking no medications.

The EEG is recorded with the patient awake following overnight sleep deprivation.

Questions: What is the interpretation of the finding in the left temporal region (*arrows a* and *b*)? What diagnosis does this finding support?

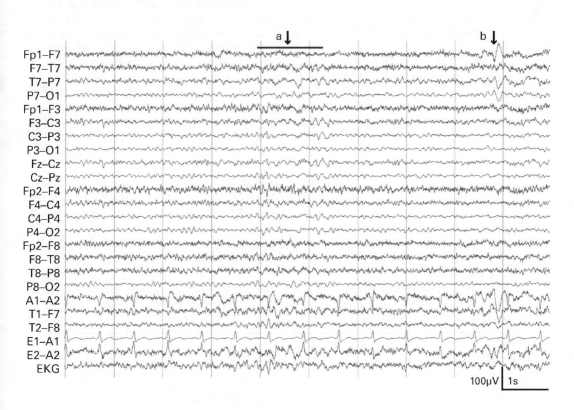

Answers: A spike (*arrow b*) localized to the left anterior temporal region and a burst of arrhythmic slowing (*arrow a*) indicate a physiologic or structural lesion of the left temporal region that is potentially epileptogenic. This finding supports a diagnosis of epileptic seizure, accounting for the patient's single episode, and implies a risk of further seizures.

Discussion: The clinical presentation of a single, new-onset seizure is one of the most common problems facing the electroencephalographer and neurologist. IEDs and epileptic seizures maintain a robust but not absolute correlation.

The sensitivity of a single routine EEG in the yield of IEDs in known epilepsy is approximately 50%. Repeating routine studies increases sensitivity but with gradually diminishing returns, eventually attaining 80–85% after the fourth recording.

The specificity of IEDs depends on the surveyed population. For example, in adults with transient loss of consciousness from either syncope or seizure, IEDs were specific for seizure in 95%. On the other hand, epileptiform activity appears in 0.4–0.5% of adults and 1.5–3.5% of children without seizures or other neurologic disorders.

The clinical import of finding IEDs in asymptomatic individuals is controversial, especially in determining work-related risks. For example, in studies of military aircrew, subjects with IEDs on screening EEG developed epilepsy at an incidence not much different to that of the base population (~2%). On the other hand, other studies calculate risks of developing epilepsy in this supernormal population at ~25%.

The clinical significance of IEDs in patients with suspected seizure, however, is much clearer. EEG helps establish the type of seizure and epilepsy syndrome, which are important for prognosis and treatment. Seizure etiology and EEG findings are the strongest predictors of seizure recurrence in adults. Meta-analyses across many studies show that, for all adults, risk of recurrent seizures following an initial, unprovoked seizure is ~40%. The risk is highest for those with a presumptive symptomatic cause and EEG findings consistent with focal abnormalities: 65%.

The variable sensitivity of IEDs in patients, on the other hand, indicates that a lack of IEDs should not be taken as evidence against seizures. In these subjects, repeated study following sleep deprivation and containing sleep should be performed. Recordings performed soon after the event in question are more likely to show IEDs.

In the present case, neuroimaging revealed no abnormalities. Based on findings of left temporal spikes and slowing, the primary neurologist recommended treatment with anticonvulsant medication for presumptive localization-related epilepsy and risk of recurrent seizures of >50%. The patient elected to not take anticonvulsant medications and not drive for her state's proscribed duration. Carbamazepine was started after a second seizure occurred 2 months after this tracing.

Clinical Pearls

1. The sensitivity of IEDs in known epilepsy is about 50% for a single study and about 80–85% for up to four studies.

2. The specificity of IEDs in healthy adults without epilepsy is controversial, but in highly selected individuals, the risk of subsequent seizures appears no greater than the base population.

3. The specificity of IEDs in subjects with suspected seizures is high and depends on the study group. The risk of recurrent seizures in adults with suspected symptomatic causes and accompanied by focal abnormalities on the EEG is ~65%.

REFERENCES

1. Berg AT, Shinnar S: The risk of seizure recurrence following a first unprovoked seizure: A quantitative review. Neurology 1991; 41(7):965–972.
2. Gotman J, Marciani MG: Electroencephalographic spiking activity, drug levels, and seizure occurrence in epileptic patients. Ann Neurol 1985; 17(6):597–603.
3. Gregory RP, Oates T, Merry RT: Electroencephalogram epileptiform abnormalities in candidates for aircrew training. Electroencephalogr Clin Neurophysiol 1993; 86(1):75–77.
4. Hendriksen IJ, Elderson A: The use of EEG in aircrew selection. Aviat Space Environ Med 2001; 72(11):1025–1033.

5. Hoefnagels W, Padberg G, Overweg J, et al: Syncope or seizure? The diagnostic value of the EEG and hyperventilation test in transient loss of consciousness. J Neurol Neurosurg Psychiatry 1991; 54(11):953–956.
6. Salinsky M, Kanter R, Dasheiff RM: Effectiveness of multiple EEGs in supporting the diagnosis of epilepsy: An operational curve. Epilepsia 1987; 28:331–334.

PATIENT 54

A 6-year-old boy after a single generalized convulsion

A 6-year-old, previously healthy boy has a generalized convulsion while walking with his mother. He has no epilepsy risk factors, such as febrile convulsions, head trauma, or CNS infection. Family history is unremarkable, and neurologic examination is normal. He is taking no medications.

The EEG is recorded with the patient awake following overnight sleep deprivation. The sample is reformatted in bipolar longitudinal, referential, and transverse bipolar montages.

Questions: Describe the location and polarity of the spikes. What diagnosis for the patient's spell do these findings support?

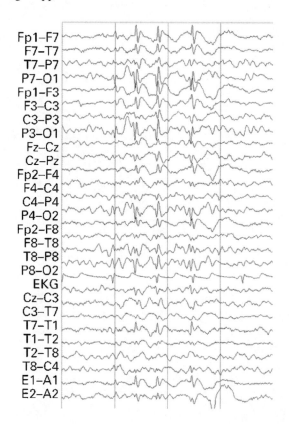

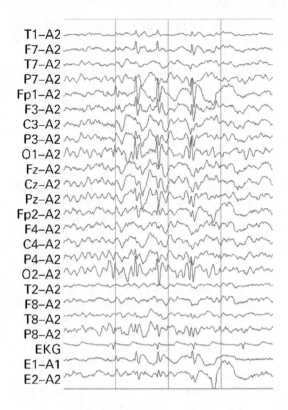

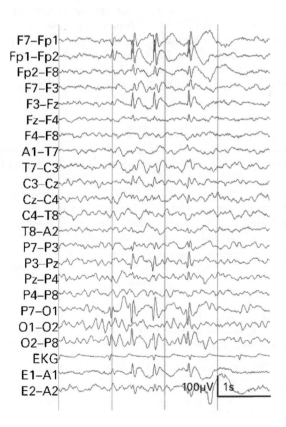

Answers: High-amplitude spikes (125–150 μV) have a morphology resembling Rolandic spikes. In the longitudinal montage, they appear with negativity at end of chain beyond Fp1 and O1 and O2. Negative phase reversal is apparent at F3, and possible positive phase reversals are apparent at C3 and P3. In the referential montage, maximum amplitudes are apparent at Fp1 and O1/O2. In the transverse view, negative phase reversals appear both at Fp1 and at O1/O2. The pattern in most consistent with a broad negativity deep within the left hemisphere with a projected, vertically oriented positive dipole. The spikes are epileptogenic but do not fall within any clear epilepsy syndrome. Although supportive of a diagnosis of epileptic seizure, the risk of seizure recurrence is unclear, despite the definitive findings of IEDs.

Discussion: The single seizure during childhood presents a different combination of challenges than that during adulthood. First, unlike adult syndromes, many childhood epilepsy syndromes are self-limited in course. Second, the social and economic effects of seizures in children are arguably less harmful than in adults. Third, children may be more susceptible to the cognitive effects of anticonvulsant medications than adults. These factors make some pediatric neurologists more likely to defer treatment with anticonvulsant medications until seizures clearly appear recurrent.

In support of this strategy are studies that find that IEDs during childhood have a less strong association with epilepsy. For example, the incidence of IEDs in healthy adults is about 0.4–0.5%, whereas the incidence is threefold or greater (1.5–3.5%) in healthy children.

Nevertheless, children with IEDs on EEG have a twofold relative risk of seizure recurrence after a first seizure than children without IEDs. EEG findings are most helpful when they help establish an epilepsy syndrome. For example, children with presumed idiopathic and cryptogenic syndromes have a 30–50% rate of recurrence of seizures within 2 years, whereas those with "remote symptomatic causes" (history of brain insult, such as mental retardation or cerebral palsy) have a >50% chance of recurrence.

In this case, spikes were present during both wakefulness and sleep. Although the spikes in this case have a morphology reminiscent of Rolandic spikes and a dipole, they are atypical from those seen in benign Rolandic epilepsy because of their basal location and persistence in all states; Rolandic spikes appear in centrotemporal regions preferentially during drowsiness. Similarly, the frontal and leftward electrical fields of the current spikes are atypical for benign occipital lobe epilepsy of childhood. Also, the spikes do not appear to emanate from a clear epileptic lesion. In the current case, therefore, no particular epilepsy syndrome is apparent. The primary neurologist for this patient recommended "expectant observation" rather than treatment with anticonvulsant medications.

Clinical Pearls

1. The incidence of IEDs in healthy children (1.5–3.5%) is higher than that of older age groups (~0.5%).

2. The adage "treat the patient, not the EEG" is most wisely followed in children; findings of IEDs in children must be placed in the context of risk and benefit.

3. Viewing selected findings with different montages, feasible with most digital EEG systems, is recommended for accurate localization.

REFERENCES

1. Berg AT, Shinnar S: The risk of seizure recurrence following a first unprovoked seizure: A quantitative review. Neurology 1991; 41(7):965–972.
2. Camfield C, Camfield P, Gordon K, Dooley J: Does the number of seizures before treatment influence ease of control or remission of childhood epilepsy? Not if the number is 10 or less. Neurology 1996; 46(1):41–44.
3. Cavazzuti GB, Cappella L, Nalin A: Longitudinal study of epileptiform EEG patterns in normal children. Epilepsia 1980; 21(1):43–45.
4. Eeg-Olofsson O, Petersen I: The development of the EEG in normal children from the age of 1 to 15 years: Paroxysmal activity. Neuropadiatrie 1971; 4:375–404.
5. Hirtz D, Berg A, Bettis D, et al: Practice parameter: Treatment of the child with a first unprovoked seizure: Report of the Quality Standards Subcommittee of the American Academy of Neurology the Practice Committee of the Child Neurology Society. Neurology 2003; 60(2):166–175.

PATIENT 55

A 3-year-old boy after a febrile convulsion

An EEG is requested to evaluate possible ongoing seizure in a 3-year-old boy who has recurrence of febrile convulsions first experienced 13 months prior. Unlike previous episodes that occurred with tympanic or rectal temperatures exceeding 38.5°C, rectal temperature during the current episode is 38°C. The patient takes no medications.

The recording is performed with the patient intermittently agitated and lethargic. Eye leads are not placed because of the agitated state.

Questions: Beyond diffuse slowing inappropriate for waking state, what is the other abnormality shown in this sample? Does the abnormality help in prognosis of epilepsy?

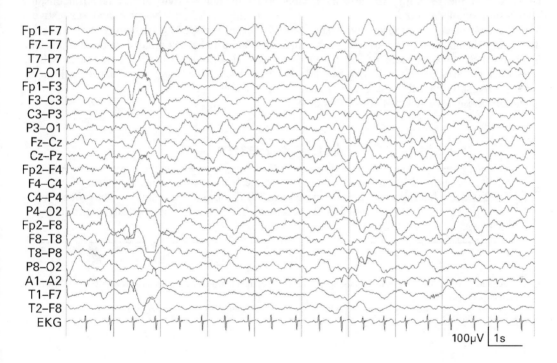

Answers: Arrhythmic delta activity is broadly distributed but focal delta activity appears in the left posterior temporal region. Localized abnormalities seen after seizure or postictal slowing are evidence of focal neuronal dysfunction. Although nonepileptiform abnormalities are associated with higher risk of afebrile seizure occurrence, epileptiform abnormalities represent a higher risk.

Discussion: *Simple febrile convulsions* are generalized seizures triggered by fever that is not due to CNS infection. Peak incidence occurs around age 18 months and is unusual past 3 years.

Complex or atypical febrile convulsions, in contrast to simple febrile convulsions, are prolonged (>30 minutes) or have partial, rather than generalized, features.

In the case of simple febrile convulsions, the EEG offers little diagnostic information. Diffuse, often occipitally dominant postictal slowing may be evident if the recording is performed soon after resolution of the seizure.

In the case of atypical febrile convulsions, or those convulsions that occur without a definite fever, the EEG may be more useful. Studies of new-onset seizures in children (not just febrile convulsions) show that the risk of recurrence is highest in those with IEDs on EEG (about two times those without abnormalities on EEG). The risk of recurrence is only marginally higher than those with normal EEGs if the abnormality is nonepileptiform (~1.3 times). However, the risk of recurrence of febrile convulsions appears to be most strongly linked to characteristics of the fever than to seizure type or electrographic findings. An increased risk of recurrent seizures is associated with a short duration of fever and a relatively lower maximum temperature.

In the present case, the predominance of arrhythmic delta activity across the left hemisphere was interpreted as abnormal and suggestive of localized nonspecific pathology. Repeat recordings are usually recommended to see if presumed focal abnormalities persist. Later cases will further discuss the appearance and significance of focal slowing.

Clinical Pearls

1. The use of EEG in the evaluation of simple febrile convulsions is unclear.
2. Focal abnormalities or IEDs in atypical febrile convulsions and other new-onset seizures in children are associated with a higher risk of spontaneously recurrent seizures.

REFERENCES

1. Berg A, Hauser W, Alemany M, et al: A prospective study of recurrent febrile seizures [see comments]. N Engl J Med 1992; 327(16):1122–1127.
2. Berg AT, Shinnar S: The risk of seizure recurrence following a first unprovoked seizure: A quantitative review. Neurology 1991; 41(7):965–972.

PATIENT 56

An 8-year-old girl with acquired aphasia and generalized convulsions

An 8-year-old girl has a 1-year history of progressive behavioral difficulties and, more recently, worsening receptive aphasia. Occasional generalized tonic-clonic seizures started about a year prior. She is treated with valproate.

The recording is performed with the patient awake.

Questions: What is the location of the spikes in the tracing? What epilepsy syndrome does this likely represent?

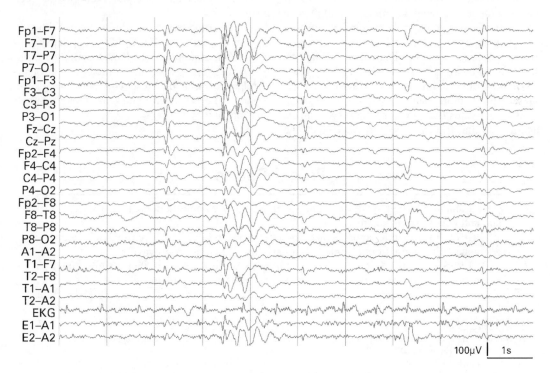

Answers: Spikes have maximum negativity in posterior temporal and central regions, with a single generalized burst of spike-wave. The clinical and electrographic findings are consistent with Landau-Kleffner syndrome.

Discussion: *Landau-Kleffner syndrome* is a rare syndrome with striking features of childhood onset of acquired aphasia and epileptic seizures or an EEG showing IEDs. Psychiatric abnormalities may be present and, in some cases, resemble autism. Receptive, rather than expressive, aphasia predominates. Generalized seizures tend to be less dramatic and more easily treated than behavioral or language abnormalities. Landau-Kleffner syndrome is usually associated with focal spikes from centroparietotemporal regions.

The broader term *epileptic aphasia* encompasses a range of related disorders that all present with various severities of behavioral abnormalities, language regression, and epilepsy. *Electrical status epilepticus of sleep* (ESES), sometimes referred to as *continuous spike-wave of slow wave sleep*, is an EEG finding of spike-wave discharges present during more than 85% of slow wave sleep.

Sleep activates IEDs in all of these syndromes, and the waking EEG can be normal. In fact, the example shown here is unusual in that the characteristic IEDs are evident during wakefulness and sleep. Because of the symptomatic overlap with autism, many centers are asked to perform EEGs as part of the evaluation of autism. If the initial daytime recording is normal and epileptic aphasia is still suspected, an overnight recording as an inpatient or with the use of outpatient ambulatory EEG should be performed to capture an adequate sample of slow wave sleep. Admittedly, the behavioral challenges present in these children sometimes make adequate sampling of sleep difficult.

Lately, some report that rare patients with syndromes similar to benign childhood epilepsy with centrotemporal spikes (Rolandic epilepsy) progress to epileptic aphasia. Although centrotemporal spikes can be present in both groups, no reports have yet determined what predictive factors may exist.

Clinical Pearls

1. Landau-Kleffner syndrome consists of psychiatric abnormalities, receptive aphasia, and generalized seizures.

2. IEDs in epileptic aphasia are activated by, and may be confined to, sleep; adequate EEG evaluation of epileptic aphasia must include slow-wave sleep.

3. ESES consists of continuous runs of spike-wave discharges that occupy slow-wave sleep and is one of the findings in syndromes of epileptic aphasia.

REFERENCES
1. Fejerman N, Caraballo R, Tenembaum SN: Atypical evolutions of benign localization-related epilepsies in children: Are they predictable? Epilepsia 2000; 41:380–390.
2. Landau WM, Kleffner FR: Syndrome of acquired aphasia with convulsive disorder in children. Neurology 1957; 7:523–530.
3. Tassinari CA, Rubboli G, Volpi L, et al: Encephalopathy with electrical status epilepticus during slow sleep or ESES syndrome including the acquired aphasia. Clin Neurophysiol 2000; 111:S94–S102.

PATIENT 57

A 24-year-old man with a right occipital cystic lesion and right mesial temporal lobe epilepsy

A 24-year-old man has medically intractable complex partial seizures with auras. He has dual pathology of a hamartoma in the right occipital lobe and right hippocampal sclerosis. Scalp video-EEG during evaluation for epilepsy surgery discloses independent, bitemporal seizure onsets, with symptoms preceding electrographic changes by more than 30 seconds. Because it is unclear whether seizures arose from the occipital lesion and spread to temporal regions or whether temporal regions served as primary epileptic foci, the patient undergoes intracranial monitoring.

The serial samples show one of the patient's typical auras of gastric lifting that does not develop into a full complex partial seizure. The patient is awake and signals an aura by pushing an event button. The montage shows intracranial electrodes in the top channels and scalp electrodes in the bottom (intrahippocampal depth electrodes [LHD, RHD]; lesional depth electrode [RPD]; subdural electrodes left frontal [LFS]; subdural electrodes left temporal [LTS]; left occipital [LOS]; right frontal [RFS]; right temporal [RTS]; right occipital [ROS]).

Questions: What is the ictal discharge? What class seizure is this event?

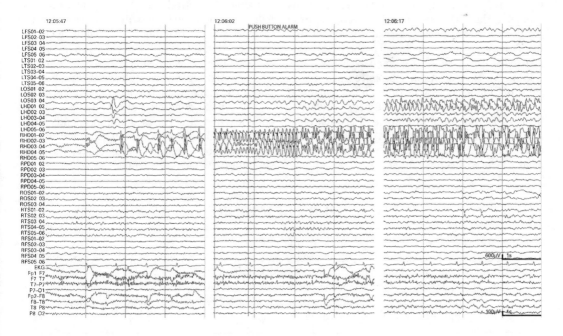

Answers: This ictal discharge consists of bursts of rhythmic spikes (first sample) at contact RHD3 (right hippocampal depth electrode). It evolved to rhythmic alpha frequency spikes (second sample) that then slowed to rhythmic theta frequencies (third sample) before slowing further to delta activities before terminating, leaving postictal slowing and suppression within the right hippocampus. The scalp EEG during discharge shows eye movement artifact (first and second samples) and some nonspecific theta slowing (third sample). The ictal discharge briefly spread to the left hippocampus (LHD, third sample). This is a simple partial seizure, an ictal discharge that does not involve enough brain to impair consciousness.

Discussion: An *ictal discharge* is any paroxysmal, rhythmic EEG activity that interrupts ongoing background activities. Ictal discharges typically evolve in frequency, amplitude, and morphology. Ictal discharges designate epileptic seizures, and, if accompanied by clinical symptoms, are diagnostic for epileptic seizures.

A *simple partial seizure* is an event limited to "simple" or single symptoms that do not affect enough brain to impair consciousness. *Auras* are warning symptoms that often precede complex partial seizures. Recordings of seizures with the use of simultaneous scalp and intracranial electrodes show that auras are merely simple partial seizures that often spare scalp electrodes. These findings are important because lack of ictal changes recorded on the scalp when consciousness is unimpaired does not rule out the possibility of an epileptic seizure.

Voltage of the discharge, the degree of synchrony among neurons involved in its generation, its location and orientation, and the affected surface area all govern the appearance of a cortical potential on the scalp. Earlier modeling experiments estimated that 20–70% of spikes recorded from the cortex never appear on scalp electrodes and that at least 6 cm^2 (about 1 square inch) of cortex is needed to generate a potential that will be "seen" by scalp electrodes. More recent comparisons of simultaneously recorded intracranial and scalp electrodes in epilepsy surgery candidates demonstrate that 90% of cortical IEDs that emanate from source areas >10 cm^2 reach the scalp. Only 10% of cortical IEDs from smaller cortical areas produced scalp potentials.

Despite their apparent accuracy, use of intracranial electrodes is limited to the localization of epileptic foci and to cortical mapping of brain functions. This is not only because of the expense and potential morbidity of an invasive procedure, but also because of the electrical properties of intracranial electrodes. Intracranial electrodes are placed upon or within cortical generators. The small conductive surface of intracranial electrodes results in high impedances. The combination of large signal and large impedances ensures that small sensitivities are required to prevent "clipping" or distortion of the display signal (note the difference in calibration bars between intracranial and scalp recordings in the previous example). Finally, the intensity of electrical fields drops with the square of the distance from the electrical source. The result of these three factors is that intracranial electrodes record from a restricted field; one pair of electrodes may record totally different activities than an immediately adjacent pair.

The implication of the limitations inherent in intracranial electrodes is that a great foreknowledge of where seizures will occur is needed in epilepsy surgery planning. Intracranial electrodes cannot be used for diagnosis of nonepileptic pseudoseizures, because the lack of electrographic seizures can be always attributed to electrode placement rather than to a nonepileptic condition.

This patient continued to have both auras and complex partial seizures that consistently arose from the right hippocampus. Right anterior temporal lobectomy significantly improved the intensity and frequency of seizures.

Clinical Pearls

1. Auras are functionally simple partial seizures.
2. Because simple partial seizures spare consciousness, and auras and simple partial seizures may not appear on scalp recordings, a normal EEG during an aura or simple partial seizure does not rule out the possibility of epileptic seizures.
3. Intracranial recordings are used for localization before some cases of epilepsy surgery and for cortical mapping of brain function.

REFERENCES

1. Abraham K, Ajmone-Marsen C: Patterns of cortical discharges and their relation to scalp EEG. Electroencephalogr Clin Neurophysiol 1958; 10:447–461.
2. Cooper R, Winter A, Crow H, Walter W: Comparison of subcortical and scalp activity using chronically indwelling electrodes in man. Electroencephalogr Clin Neurophysiol 1965; 18:217–228.
3. Tao JX, Ray A, Hiawes-Ebersole JS, Ebersole JS: Intracranial EEG substrates of scalp EEG interictal spikes. Epilepsia 2005; 46:667–676.

PATIENT 58

A 39-year-old man with frequent spells of right face twitching and tremulousness

A 39-year-old man has recent-onset spells of diffuse tremulousness and loss of consciousness. He is currently taking phenytoin.

The recording was a baseline before diagnostic intensive monitoring with video-EEG. Sequential 4-second samples are shown. The technologist asks him questions when she notes the onset of electrographic activity, and the patient responds normally. No motor symptoms are seen.

Question: What is the diagnosis of the activity?

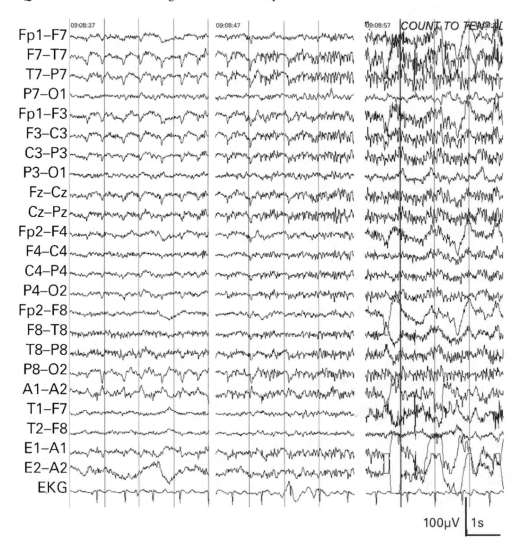

Answer: *Subclinical rhythmic electrographic discharge in adults* (SREDA). The finding is not a seizure and is not associated with epilepsy.

Discussion: SREDA is a benign, rhythmic pattern. Although rare, it is important to recognize because it is a rhythmic activity that can be mistaken for an epileptic seizure.

Location. The distribution of rhythmic activity is usually diffuse with temporal predominance.

Morphology. SREDA consists of the abrupt appearance of rhythmic, monophasic, sharply contoured activities that progressively occur at shorter intervals, usually in the theta frequency band. The progression from slow to fast frequencies is helpful in its distinction from most epileptic ictal discharges, because the latter may evolve from faster to slower frequencies.

Reactivity/state. It occurs in adults during restful wakefulness or drowsiness. SREDA is the exception to many benign epileptiform transients because it usually occurs during wakefulness.

Patients have no symptoms during SREDA. Unlike many ictal discharges, there is no postictal slowing of the tracing following resolution.

This patient reported none of his typical symptoms during the discharge during the sample. He did, however, experience several of his typical spells during intensive video-EEG. Events featured preserved alpha rhythm during apparent unresponsiveness, a finding not consistent with encephalopathy or ongoing epileptic seizure. His diagnosis was psychogenic nonepileptic pseudoseizures.

Clinical Pearls

1. SREDA is a benign, subclinical burst of rhythmic activity seen in adults that can be distinguished from ictal discharges by its lack of clinical accompaniment and its evolution atypical from seizures.

2. Direct diagnosis of seizures requires the recording of the patient's typical symptomatology during EEG. Events atypical for the complaints at hand may not predict etiology of chronic, recurrent spells.

REFERENCE

1. Westmoreland B, Klass D: A distinctive, rhythmic EEG discharge of adults. Electroencephalogr Clin Neurophysiol 1981; 51:186–189.

PATIENT 59

A 53-year-old man with intractable epilepsy undergoing intensive video-EEG

A 53-year-old man has a 20-year history of medically intractable complex partial seizures and has suspected mesial temporal lobe epilepsy (MTLE).

The patient is awake during this recording and eating. Anticonvulsant medications have been withdrawn.

Questions: What is the bitemporal rhythmic activity during the first third of the sample? From what region does the seizure arise? Referring to the times at the top of the tracing, how long after clinical onset does electrographic onset of his typical complex partial seizure begin?

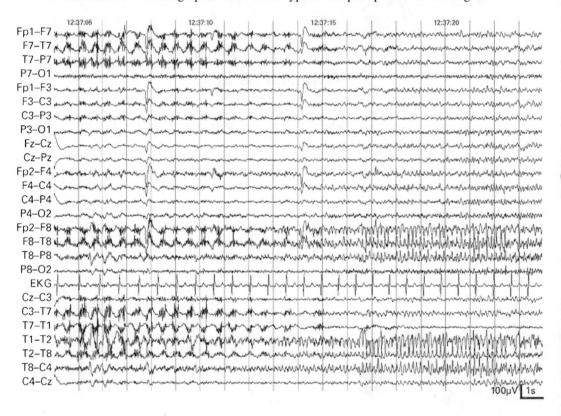

Answers: The bitemporal rhythmic activity during the first third of the sample is chewing artifact. The seizure arises from the right anterior-temporal region. Clinical onset occurs at 12:37:14, corresponding to cessation of ongoing waking activities (cessation of chewing artifact, eating lunch). Electrographic onset, marked by emergence of rhythmic fast activities, occurs around 12:37:11. Electrode T8 appears to be the earliest electrode involved, with rhythmic 7 cps sharp theta activity appearing with maximum negativity at electrodes F8 and T2 immediately after onset. This seizure arises from the right side, with best localization to the right anterior-midtemporal region. Electrographic onset precedes clinical onset by ~3 seconds.

Discussion: Ictal discharges from focal epileptic lesions can assume various morphologies when recorded from the scalp, depending on such factors as location, depth, and surface area involved. Two typical patterns are

1. Focal attenuation, low-amplitude rhythmic, sharp, fast activity between 10 and 30 cps that gradually builds in amplitude and decreases in frequency
2. Progression of rhythmic spikes or spike-wave complexes that build up in frequency before evolving to higher-amplitude, slow-frequency spikes or spike-wave complexes.

Following resolution of the ictal discharge, postictal suppression or slowing can be diffuse or more severe from the originating site.

In the presurgical evaluation of subjects with MTLE, several features of the ictal discharge recorded from the scalp correlate well with the gold standard of localization with the use of hippocampal depth electrodes:

1. Electrographic onset before emergence of clear clinical symptoms is reassuring. The reverse sequence—clinical onset before electrographic onset—implies that seizures may arise from an unseen focus before late seizure activity arises on the scalp.
2. Focal development of anterior temporal rhythmic theta or alpha spike activity (>5 cps) is one of the strongest localizing signs in scalp recordings of MTLE patients.
3. Ictal discharges that remain confined to one region, or at least remain unilateral for at least 5 seconds before spreading contralaterally, are good evidence of focal onset.
4. Focal postictal slowing is a reliable indicator of side of seizure onset, but the finding is present in the minority of scalp recordings of patients with MTLE. Many show diffuse postictal slowing.

Concordant findings among scalp IEDs, scalp ictal recordings, neuroimaging, and neuropsychological testing predict excellent results (80–90% seizure-free outcome in some series) from anterior temporal lobectomy or selective amygdala-hippocampectomy in patients with MTLE.

Clinical Pearls

1. Important localizing features of ictal scalp recordings in patients with MTLE include (1) electrographic onset of focal ictal changes before clinical onset; (2) development of a unilateral, focal ictal discharge consisting of rhythmic theta or alpha activity; (3) confinement of the ictal discharge to one hemisphere for at least 5 seconds before contralateral spread; and (4) focal postictal slowing.

2. Bitemporal bursts of rhythmic muscle activity arise from chewing artifact.

REFERENCES

1. Risinger MW, Engel J, Van Ness PC, et al: Ictal localization of temporal lobe seizures with scalp/sphenoidal recordings. Neurology 1989; 39:1288–1293.
2. Williamson P, French J, Thadani V, et al: Characteristics of medial temporal lobe epilepsy. II: Interictal and ictal scalp electroencephalography, neuropsychological testing, neuroimaging, surgical results, and pathology. Ann Neurol 1993; 34(6):781–787.

PATIENT 60

A 30-year-old woman with spells

A 30-year-old woman is evaluated for epilepsy that did not respond to treatment with phenytoin or carbamazepine. Seizures started 1 year prior after a motor vehicle accident in which she had a minor concussion and two family members were killed.

The sample is taken during intensive monitoring with video-EEG. The monitor watcher pushes the event button when the patient ceases speaking to another patient, stares, begins facial grimacing, and is unresponsive to her roommate or the monitor-watcher's interview over the intercom.

Question: Does the tracing provide evidence of epileptic seizure?

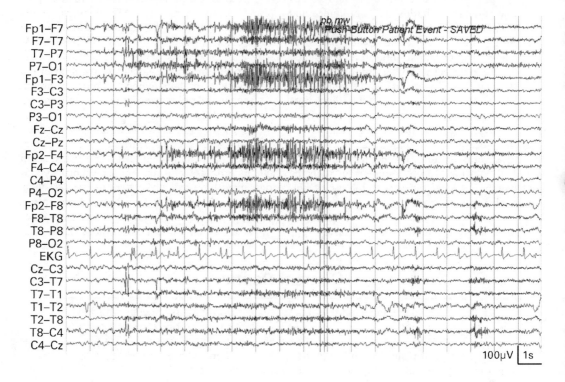

Answer: No. The tracing shows bursts of muscle activity that often obscure cerebral activity. Posterior rhythms of wakefulness can be discerned intermittently during the spell. This recording is most consistent with a nonepileptic pseudoseizure.

Discussion: This example shows evidence of normal ongoing activities of wakefulness despite clinical unresponsiveness. This recording was corroborated by several other events that featured preserved alpha rhythm during apparent unresponsiveness, a finding not consistent with encephalopathy or ongoing seizure. It is a key observation in the diagnosis of *psychogenic nonepileptic pseudoseizures* (PNES).

Clues to diagnosis of PNES are unrecognized depression, anxiety, dissociative traits, or posttraumatic stress disorder. A history of acute stressors can help in the diagnosis of conversion disorder. Patients with PNES have high incidences of sexual or physical abuse.

Spells of PNES frequently last longer than the 1–2 minutes of typical complex partial seizures. Spells of PNES may wax and wane in intensity compared to the monophasic course of complex partial seizures. Despite these differences, elaborateness or peculiarity of behaviors is not predictive of PNES, because complex partial seizures of frontal lobe origin are notorious for bizarre symptomatology.

Confirmatory monitoring with the use of intensive video-EEG is usually required for diagnosis. Not only do the various symptoms seen in each disease overlap, but comorbidity of pseudoseizures and epileptic seizures ranges from 25–75% depending upon study methods.

Clinical examination during intensive EEG monitoring is an important part of the diagnosis.

Determination of the degree of impairment during spells may facilitate their proper classification. The table below summarizes possible results from the well-conducted diagnostic intensive monitoring session:

Clinical Impairment	Ictal Discharge	
	Yes	No
Yes	Epileptic seizure	Pseudoseizure
No	Electrographic seizure	Simple partial seizure Pseudoseizure

Circumstances exist in which seizures do not appear on scalp recordings. Muscle or movement artifact may obscure the EEG; clues, such as initial focal slowing or IEDs or postictal slowing, may then be helpful. Partial seizures may not involve a critical amount of brain or may arise from deeper cortical areas and remain occult. Sixteen percent of complex partial seizures confirmed by intracranial electrode recordings may not appear on scalp recordings. In cases in which scalp recordings are unclear or obscured, stereotypy of patient's behaviors during repeated events may be the only recourse to suggest an epileptic cause. Prolactin levels, a pituitary hormone that undergoes acute elevation after complex partial seizures, may aid in diagnosis in selected cases.

Clinical Pearls

1. Psychogenic nonepileptic seizures require the capturing of typical spells on EEG to make a positive diagnosis because the clinical characteristics and comorbidities between nonepileptic and epileptic seizures are high.

2. Alteration of consciousness with preservation of alpha rhythm and other waking activities is characteristic of nonepileptic pseudoseizures captured on EEG.

3. Events without alteration of consciousness or during which consciousness is not determined may have ambiguous conclusions during EEG monitoring.

REFERENCES

1. Devinsky O: Nonepileptic psychogenic seizures: Quagmires of pathophysiology, diagnosis, and treatment. Epilepsia 1998; 39:458–462.
2. Gates JR, Ramani V, Whalen S, Loewenson R: Ictal characteristics of pseudoseizures. Arch Neurol 1985; 42:1183–1187.
3. Pacia SV, Ebersole JS: Intracranial EEG substrates of scalp ictal patterns from temporal lobe foci. Epilepsia 1997; 38(6):642–654.

PATIENT 61

A 2-day-old term infant with right body clonus

A 2-day-old term infant (ECA 40 weeks) is born in respiratory distress. Meconium staining is present. Serum sodium is low at 126 mg/dL. Right body clonus is observed by nursing staff shortly after birth. Medications are ampicillin and gentamicin.

The recording is performed with routine neonatal polygraphy at the bedside. No age-appropriate activities are seen; instead, unreactive burst-suppression is present throughout the recording. No clinical seizures occurred during the tracing.

Question: What is the activity in the left temporal region?

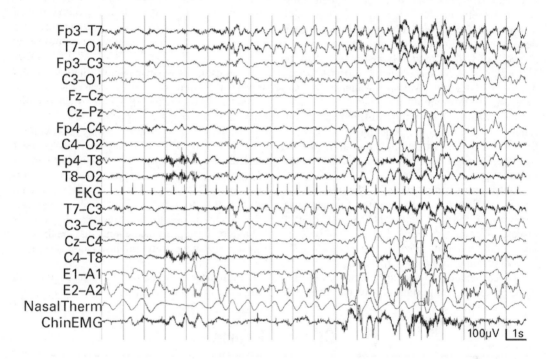

Answer: Left temporal focal seizure.

Discussion: The main challenge in evaluating neonatal seizures is the distinction of clinical seizures from nonepileptic, stereotypic, and repetitive movements. A second challenge is the identification of electrographic seizures, a task made more difficult because of properties of the immature brain.

Because of incomplete connections within and between cortex and subcortical structures, neonates are unable to sustain generalized electrographic seizures. Instead, clonic, multifocal clonic, and tonic seizures occur that involve groups of muscles in a migratory or asymmetric fashion. Motor automatisms, such as "jitteriness," bicycling, repetitive sucking or orofacial movements, or apnea, are behaviors that are observed frequently in ill infants and usually do not correspond to ictal discharges. Nevertheless, often the EEG is required to supplement clinical observation.

Ictal discharges can take several different patterns based on frequency and morphology, but specific patterns correlate poorly with specific causes or outcome. Ictal patterns can consist of (1) rhythmic runs of spikes, (2) sharply contoured slow waves or epileptiform complexes, or (3) runs of rhythmic activity of changing frequency and morphology. Each kind can remain in one region, migrate from one region to another, or arise in an independent, multifocal pattern. As a rule, however, neonatal electrographic seizures do not generalize.

Two features make recognition of neonatal electrographic seizures difficult. The first is that ictal discharges may involve only one electrode and thereby be attributed mistakenly to artifact. The second is that waveforms may remain monomorphic and occur at a slow rhythm, 0.25–1 cps, in some cases. Because the eye becomes trained to ignore very slow activities reminiscent of movement or galvanic artifacts, potential seizures can be easily missed. One technique to emphasize "latent" evolution of morphology and frequency typical of ictal discharges is to decrease the paper speed to compress slow wave activities.

The prognosis of neonatal seizures lies with the underlying cause. Electrographic seizures without clinical accompaniment and invariant, age-discordant background activities indicate poor prognosis of normal intellectual development.

Clinical Pearls

1. Neonatal seizures often consist of monomorphic, focal runs of rhythmic activity that, although often migratory or multifocal, do not generalize.

2. Recognition of neonatal seizures after initial screening with standard paper speed can be augmented by review of suspicious rhythmic activities with slow paper speed.

REFERENCES

1. McBride MC, Laroia N, Guillet R: Electrographic seizures in neonates correlate with poor neurodevelopmental outcome. Neurology 2000; 55(4):506–513.
2. Mizrahi EM, Kellaway P: Characterization and classification of neonatal seizures. Neurology 1987; 37:1837–1844.

PATIENT 62

A 1-week-old male infant with apnea

A 1-week-old male infant, born at estimated gestational age 39 weeks, presents with a right parenchymal hemorrhage and apneic spells. The infant is treated with phenobarbital.

The 30-second sample is taken from routine neonatal polygraphy at the bedside during quiet sleep. Electrographic seizure activity, in the form of rhythmic spike activity starting in the right frontocentrotemporal region and evolving to right centrotemporal delta activity, starts about 10 seconds before the sample.

Questions: What is the finding in the respiratory (nasal thermosister) channel? Is there a significant change in heart rate accompanying the seizure?

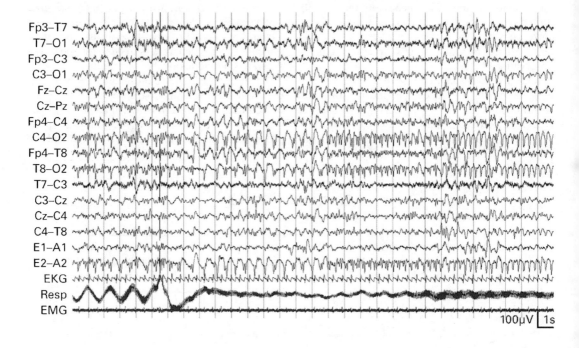

Answers: The lack of respiratory air flow defines apnea. No significant change in heart rate is present during this apneic seizure.

Discussion: *Apnea* in the full-term neonate is defined as a cessation of breathing for more than 20 seconds. *Obstructive apneas* are defined as those in which respiratory effort persists throughout the apnea; respiratory effort ceases in *central apneas*. *Mixed apneas* contain apneas with intermittent respiratory effort. Respiratory effort is usually measured by thoracic and abdominal strain gauges, inputs that are absent in this example.

The differential diagnosis of apnea in the newborn is broad. Apnea can arise from airway obstruction (obstructive apnea), gastroesophageal reflux, cardiopulmonary disease, or, as in this case, epileptic seizures (central or mixed apnea). Furthermore, idiopathic apnea of central or mixed origin may arise because of immaturity of brainstem and peripheral regulatory systems.

Epileptic apneas, in comparison to other causes of apnea, are relatively rare in the full-term infant and not apparent in the premature infant. Most apneas in the full-term neonate are accompanied by bradycardia, the result of over-vigorous cardio-inhibitory reflexes of the immature nervous system. Epileptic seizures, conversely, typically override any compensatory reflex activity in the newborn, so that epileptic apneas are rarely associated with bradycardia. For example, in one study of 112 apneas in 15 neonates (6 of whom were premature), epileptic apneas occurred in 4 of the full-term infants. No apneas were accompanied by bradycardia.

In this patient's case, apneas presented as the sole manifestation of epilepsy, a finding not unusual in previous studies. In the full-term neonate, epileptic seizures should be considered as potential causes of apneic events, even in the absence of other behaviors suspicious for seizures.

Clinical Pearls

1. Neonatal nonepileptic apneas typically occur with bradycardia; epileptic apnea usually occurs without bradycardia.

2. Although epileptic apnea should be considered in the full-term infant, epileptic apneas are basically unreported in the premature infant.

REFERENCES

1. Fenichel GM, Olson BJ, Fitzpatrick JE: Heart rate changes in convulsive and nonconvulsive neonatal apnea. Ann Neurol 1980; 7:577–582.
2. Tramonte JJ, Goodkin HP: Temporal lobe hemorrhage in the full-term neonate presenting as apneic seizures. J Perinatol 2004; 24:726–729.

PATIENT 63

A 1-week-old female infant with apnea

A 1-week-old female infant (born at estimated gestational age 39 weeks) presents with recurrent episodes of apnea and oxygen desaturation. Apneic spells were associated with tongue thrusting movements. Medications are famotidine.

The 30-second sample is recorded during overnight video-polygraphy with the patient asleep (eyes closed on video).

Questions: In what state is the patient during this sample? Describe the two marked episodes *(bars).*

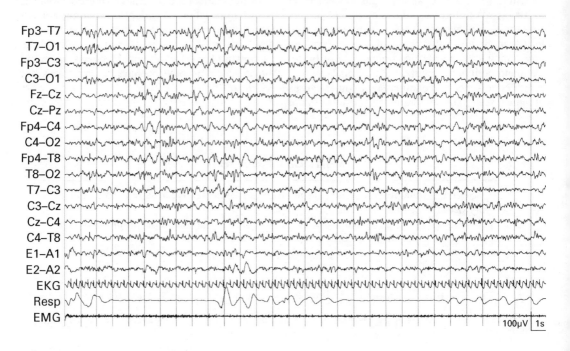

Answers: The patient is in active sleep. Brief apneas that are not accompanied by bradycardia or CNS disturbance. These are normal apneas.

Discussion: Clinically significant apneas in the neonate either exceed 20 seconds in duration, or, if briefer, are accompanied by oxygen desaturation or bradycardia. The incidence and duration of apnea increase with decreasing gestational age at birth. They normally resolve with increasing maturation; in one study, apneic spells ceased in 92% of infants by 37 weeks ECA and in 98% by 40 weeks.

Apneas typically occur during active sleep, as the brief events seen in this case.

The causes of apnea and their severity are typically divided into those affecting premature infants versus full-term infants.

This idiopathic syndrome, termed *apneas of prematurity,* results from dysregulation of the cardiopulmonary system because of immaturity of the central nervous system and peripheral baroceptor and chemoceptor responses. Diagnosis is made by identifying possible causes of secondary apnea, mainly sepsis, metabolic abnormalities, and CNS hemorrhage. Monitoring is typically limited to oxygen saturation and EKG monitors. Although clinically significant apneas typically resolve by term, subtle dysfunction, marked by brief apneas and less-rhythmic breathing, persists in infants, particularly those with small birth weights.

In term infants, epileptic seizures are an infrequent but important cause of clinically significant apnea. Epileptic apneas usually arise in conjunction with other seizure behaviors but rarely in isolation from other clinical seizure activities.

In this patient's case, overnight polygraphy captured numerous episodes of brief apneas. None were accompanied by electrographic seizure activity, and none exceeded 20 seconds in duration or were associated with desaturation. Because waking and sleep activities were appropriate for ECA and neither seizures nor IEDs were found, epileptic seizures were removed from consideration in the differential diagnosis.

Clinical Pearls

1. Brief apneas without clinical accompaniments are common in term infants.
2. Clinically significant apneas are common in premature infants, with severity and incidence inversely related to ECA.
3. Apneas are most common during active sleep.

REFERENCES

1. Curzi-Dascalova L, Peirano P, Christova E: Respiratory characteristics during sleep in healthy small-for-gestational age newborns. Pediatrics 1996; 97:554–559.
2. Henderson-Smart DJ: The effect of gestational age on the incidence and duration of recurrent apnoea in newborn babies. Aust Paediatr J 1981; 17:273–276.

PATIENT 64

A 37-year-old man with apparent complex partial seizures

An EEG is requested in a 37-year-old man with static encephalopathy and apparent recurrent complex partial seizures that has increased in occurrence since a switch to carbamazepine from an unknown anticonvulsant medication.

The EEG is recorded with the patient awake. The notations refer to response testing shown in the bottom channel. Deviations in potential are caused by the technologist pushing a button that creates an audible signal to which the patient is instructed to respond with a button of his own.

Question: Is this an interictal or ictal discharge? What type of seizure is the patient experiencing?

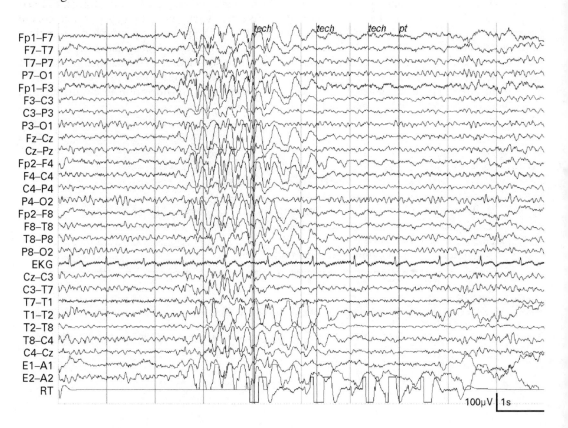

Answer: The lack of patient responses during spike-wave discharges and an intact response with resolution of the discharge confirm that this is an ictal discharge, that is, both a clinical and electrographic seizure. The sample shows rhythmic, generalized multispike-wave and spike wave discharges that occur at a rate of 2.5–3.5 cps. This discharge is more consistent with an atypical absence seizure than a complex partial seizure.

Discussion: *Atypical absence seizures* are defined as episodes of inattention, behavioral arrest, and limited motor automatisms or changes in tone. Atypical absences usually last longer than absence seizures but often occur less frequently, making them sometimes difficult to distinguish by clinical observation from complex partial seizures.

The hallmark of an atypical absence seizure is generalized spike-wave discharges. Unlike the classic 3 cps spike-wave bursts of absence seizures, frequency of occurrence is usually between 1.5 and 2.5 cps. Multiple spike-wave discharges, or a mix of spike-wave and multiple spike-wave, occur frequently. Background EEGs are usually helpful in that they are usually abnormal in those with atypical absences and usually normal in those with typical absences.

The division between interictal epileptiform discharges and clinically apparent ictal discharges is not always clear, especially in the generalized epilepsies. For example, although a myoclonic seizure may be accompanied by a generalized ictal discharge, the duration of the seizure may be too brief to accurately determine any degree of impairment. The division, however, goes beyond academic interest. Questions regarding the ability to drive, assessments of poor learning in school, and efficacy of treatment regimens often pivot on the determination if a specific discharge is accompanied by clinical impairment of consciousness or cognition.

An aid in this decision is *response testing*. As shown in the example, both the technologist and patient have similar buttons. When a discharge occurs on the EEG, the technologist can rapidly ascertain if call-and-response is impaired.

In this patient's case, the distinction between atypical absence seizures and complex partial seizures is important because these findings can direct anticonvulsant selection. The patient's medication is changed to a broad-spectrum anticonvulsant because carbamazepine, although suited for partial seizures, may exacerbate generalized seizures.

Clinical Pearls

1. Atypical absence seizures are marked by generalized spike-wave or multiple spike-wave bursts with frequencies less than 3 cps.

2. Response testing is a procedure that can distinguish between interictal and ictal activity by documenting impairment in attention and responsiveness.

REFERENCES
1. Perucca E, Gram L, Avanzini G, Dulac O: Antiepileptic drugs as a cause of worsening seizures. Epilepsia 1998; 39:5–17.

PATIENT 65

A 25-year-old man with Lennox-Gastaut syndrome and drop attacks

A 25-year-old man has Lennox-Gastaut syndrome that, until recently, was expressed with frequent generalized tonic-clonic seizures and atypical absence seizures. Over the previous 3 months, he began abruptly falling without warning. No overt seizure activity is seen before or after events.

The recording is performed with the patient awake. Medications are valproate and zonisamide. While sitting upright, the patient is observed to abruptly stiffen and slump to the floor.

Question: What type of seizure accounts for the patient's drop attacks?

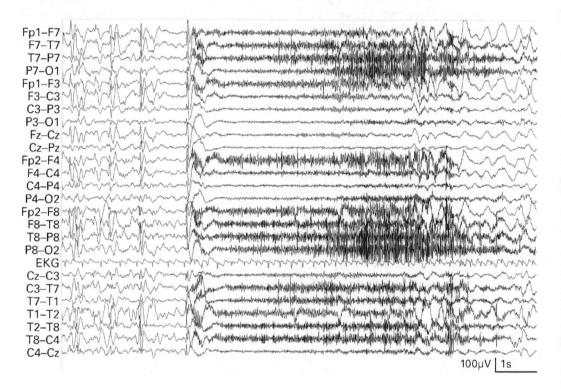

Answer: The recording is diagnostic for a tonic seizure. Generalized fast activity, appearing as diffuse attenuation, corresponds to the patient's symptoms of brief hypertonia.

Discussion: Epileptic *drop attacks* can result from generalized or rapid secondary generalization of partial seizures. *Tonic seizures*, shown here, consist of brief, generalized hypertonic episodes, sometimes called *axial spasms*. The EEG shows bursts of generalized fast activities, usually preceded by a high-amplitude, generalized spike-wave.

Tonic seizures are most commonly encountered in Lennox-Gastaut syndrome; in fact, nocturnal bursts of generalized fast activities accompanied by tonic seizures are thought by some to be pathomnemonic of Lennox-Gastaut syndrome.

Atonic seizures cause falls from abrupt generalized loss of tone. Various ictal discharges can be seen. Atonic seizures preceded by brief myoclonus are seen in the rare epileptic syndrome of childhood *myoclonic-astatic epilepsy* (Doose syndrome), differentiated from Lennox-Gastaut syndrome by its association with relatively preserved cognition, predisposition to photoparoxysmal responses, and family history.

Partial seizures can rapidly secondarily generalize and interrupt maintenance of extensor tone. So-called "temporal lobe syncope" may occur in patients with medically intractable complex partial seizures of either temporal or frontal lobe origin.

Syncope from various common cardiovascular causes, as well as rare cases of epileptic seizures that induce bradycardia or asystole, can mimic primary epileptic drop attacks. Cataplexy, in the setting of unrecognized narcolepsy, can be confusing as the cause of drop attacks until the characteristic daytime sleepiness is characterized.

Clinical Pearls

1. Tonic seizures are pathomnemonic findings in Lennox-Gastaut syndrome and consist of bursts of generalized fast activity.

2. The differential diagnosis of epileptic drop attacks includes generalized seizures and rapidly secondarily generalized seizures from frontal or temporal lobe foci. Syncope and cataplexy may present with drop attacks.

REFERENCES

1. Brenner RP, Atkinson R: Generalized paroxysmal fast activity: Electroencephalographic and clinical features. Ann Neurol 1982; 11:386–390.
2. Doose H: Myoclonic-astatic epilepsy. Epilepsy Res Suppl 1992; 6:163–168.
3. Gambardella A, Reutens D, Andermann F: Late-onset drop attacks in temporal lobe epilepsy: A reevaluation of the concept of temporal lobe syncope. Neurology 1994; 44(6):1074–1078.
4. Quigg M, Bleck T: Syncope. In Engel J, Pedley T (eds). Epilepsy: A Comprehensive Textbook. New York, Lippincott-Raven, 1997, pp 2649–2659.

PATIENT 66

A 17-month-old girl with drop attacks

A 17-month-old girl has onset of recurrent drop attacks 1 month prior. Drop attacks were usually followed by brief episodes of myoclonic jerks. The child was born at term and has normal development. Although the parents state that spells occurred spontaneously, on closer history the child was often crying before the episodes. The spells did not resolve with a trial of phenytoin.

The recording is performed with the child awake, upset, and crying. She is taking no medications.

Question: What is the etiology of the event captured during the tracing?

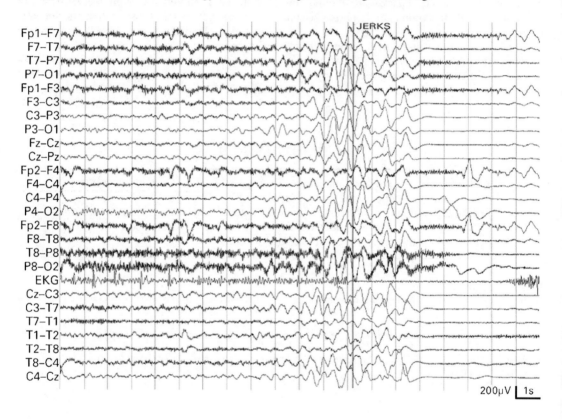

Ictal Discharges and Epileptic Seizures

Answer: The tracing shows abrupt development of generalized, semirhythmic delta activity followed by suppression coinciding with onset of symptoms. The EKG shows loss of the QRS complex before EEG changes. This recording is diagnostic for cerebral hypoperfusion caused by crying-provoked asystole (breath-holding).

Discussion: *Syncope* refers to the abrupt and transient loss of consciousness and motor tone caused by loss of cerebral perfusion. The most common causes stem from alterations of cardiovascular tone or direct cardiac dysfunction.

Breath-holding events usually occur in infants and toddlers between ages 6 and 18 months. Spells are usually triggered by crying but can also be provoked by grunting or defecation or other activities that raise intrathoracic pressure. Traditionally, spells are divided into cyanotic and pallid subtypes.

Transient cerebral hypoperfusion causes abrupt changes in the EEG. Usually, bursts of semirhythmic-to-rhythmic delta activities emerge with loss of consciousness and can be followed by suppression if lasting for more than 5–10 seconds. *Syncopal myoclonus*, sometimes termed *syncopal convulsions,* consisting of brief, generalized myoclonic jerks, is present in over 80% of cases of syncope induced in research studies. No ictal discharges accompany syncopal myoclonus.

EEG is not a useful screening tool in most cases of routine syncope. Nevertheless, EEG is called upon during evaluations of more unusual or severe cases. In this case, syncope was suspected during initial consultation because drop attacks from epileptic causes usually occur in syndromes with abnormal developmental histories, for example, tonic seizures in Lennox-Gastaut syndrome.

This child was managed conservatively at first, but spells recurred. Cardiology evaluations were normal. Finally, two severe episodes lasting over 2 minutes occurred, and her cardiologist recommended placement of a cardiac pacemaker.

Clinical Pearls

1. The EEG during syncope shows development of generalized delta activity corresponding to acute loss of consciousness. Progression to suppression may occur if cerebral hypoperfusion persists.

2. Syncopal myoclonus can be observed during many episodes of syncope and are not epileptic in origin.

3. Although EEG is not a useful screening tool in routine evaluation of syncope, in unusual cases it is a sensitive and specific technique, if a spell is captured.

REFERENCES

1. Aminoff M, Scheinman M, Griffin J, Herre J: Electrocerebral accompaniments of syncope associated with malignant ventricular arrhythmias. Ann Intern Med 1988; 108(6):791–796.
2. Quigg M, Bleck T: Syncope. In Engel J, Pedley T (eds). Epilepsy: A Comprehensive Textbook. New York, Lippincott-Raven, 1997, pp 2649–2659.

PATIENT 67

A 73-year-old woman with confusion and left hemiparesis

A 73-year-old woman is admitted with a right hemispheric intracerebral hemorrhagic stroke causing left hemiparesis. After admission, her level of consciousness declines, and repeat neuroimaging shows no evidence of progressive bleed or edema.

The patient during this recording is confused but awake. She is taking no CNS-active medications. The patient is asked to close her eyes but only flutters them in response.

Questions: What is the abnormality? What is the most likely cause?

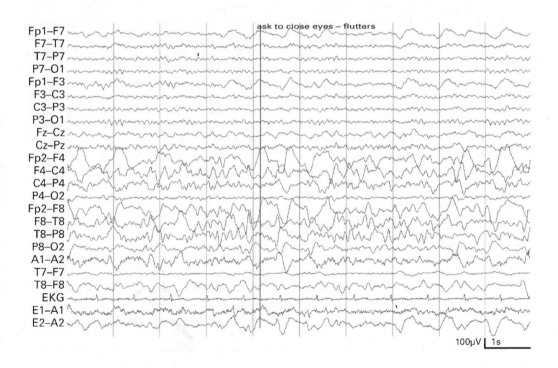

Answers: Continuous, unreactive, arrhythmic delta activity is present across right frontal-temporal-central regions. Focal arrhythmic delta activity indicates a structural lesion of the area, corresponding to the region of hemorrhagic stroke.

Discussion: At one time, EEG, neurologic examination, arteriography, and pneumoencephalography were the only means by which to determine the existence of a focal cerebral lesion in the living patient. Autopsy was often the tie-breaker in unclear cases. Currently, the neuroimaging techniques of computed tomography (CT) and magnetic resonance imaging (MRI) have largely supplanted EEG's former role in the investigation of focal lesions. MRI, for example, far exceeds the ability of EEGs to determine the presence of a focal tumor. Nevertheless, the usefulness of EEG exceeds its relatively poor sensitivity, for it currently remains the only widespread tool, outside of clinical exam, that can determine the functional consequences of a presumed lesion.

Focal lesions alter the EEG in three important ways.

1. Focal lesions may cause changes in normal activities. For example, the alpha rhythm ipsilateral to the hemisphere containing the focal lesion may demonstrate slowing in frequency, decrement in amplitude, or a defect in persistence and reactivity. Sleep activities may be poorly developed or absent on the affected side.
2. Focal lesions may cause abnormalities elicited with activation procedures. Asymmetry of photic driving suggests the presence of an ipsilateral physiologic or anatomic lesion. A similar interpretation follows focal slowing induced during hyperventilation. These physiologic changes, however, should be corroborated by other evidence of localized dysfunction.
3. Focal lesions may also cause the emergence of abnormal activities, specifically, focal theta or delta activity.

Two main morphologies of slowing are *intermittent rhythmic delta activity* (IRDA) and *arrhythmic delta activity* (ADA). IRDA appears as bursts of sinusoidal, rhythmic delta activities, usually reactive to state or stimulation, and implies physiologic rather than structural abnormalities. ADA consists of mixed low frequencies and is usually the consequence of a fixed lesion. The mixture of slow frequencies creates an appearance of ''polymorphic'' slowing.

The technologist should demonstrate whether slowing is reactive and altered or improved with patient stimulation or endogenous arousal. Although there are no clear divisions in the severity of focal slowing, more slow frequencies, greater persistence, and unreactivity correspond to more profound lesions.

Studies show that focal slowing is most reliably generated from white matter lesions that interrupt connections to and from the cortex. Tumors, strokes, and abscesses are typical causes of structural lesions. Focal slowing is a nonspecific response; therefore, physiologic lesions, such as postictal slowing from epileptogenic zones or even transient perfusion abnormalities from complicated migraine, can generate focal slowing.

Clinical Pearls

1. Focal slowing indicates localized cerebral dysfunction and most reliably occurs with disruption of the underlying white matter.
2. Focal slowing can take the form of sporadic, intermittent, or continuous slowing.
3. Intermittent rhythmic delta activity implies a physiologic lesion, and arrhythmic delta activity structural lesion, although activities are certainly not restricted to these specific interpretations.

REFERENCES

1. Gloor P, Ball G, Schaul N: Brain lesions that produce delta waves in the EEG. Neurology 1977; 27:326–333.
2. Schaul N: Pathogenesis and significance of abnormal nonepileptiform rhythms in the EEG. J Clin Neurophysiol 1990; 7:229–248.
3. Walter WG: The location of cerebral tumours by electroencephalography. Lancet 1936; 2:305–308.

PATIENT 68

A 33-year-old man with suspected mesial temporal lobe epilepsy

A 33-year-old man presents with adolescent-onset, medically refractory complex partial seizures with features suggesting the syndrome of mesial temporal lobe epilepsy (MTLE). Medications are levetiracetam and carbamazepine.

The recording is obtained with the patient awake. The sample is shown in both bipolar and referential montages. Bursts of delta activity shown here occur intermittently during the tracing.

Questions: What is the location of focal slowing? What is its clinical import?

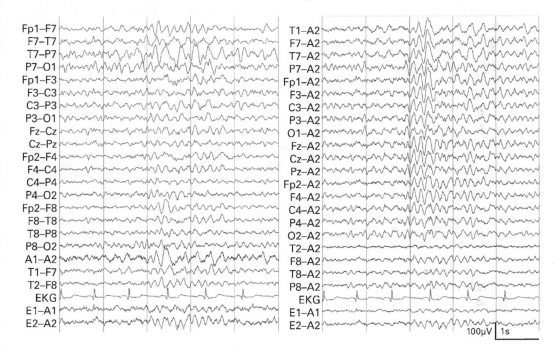

Answers: The focal slowing is *temporal intermittent rhythmic delta activity* (TIRDA), with widespread field with highest amplitudes across the temporal region. It is potentially epileptogenic.

Discussion: TIRDA occupies a special place in the hierarchy of focal delta activity. Unlike other focal slowing, a nonspecific indicator of localized cerebral pathology, TIRDA is associated with epileptogenic regions in patients with epilepsy. Thus, TIRDA is the only epileptogenic focal finding that is not epileptiform.

TIRDA consists of intermittent bursts of sinusoidal delta activities. Sharp waves or spikes are often present in the same tracing and may appear with bursts of TIRDA.

TIRDA has been usually studied in the setting of MTLE during consideration of epilepsy surgery. In this subgroup of patients, TIRDA is highly predictive of side of seizure onset and thus a finding supporting lateralization and localization. TIRDA is not limited to patients with MTLE and has been seen in patients with localization-related epilepsies not of temporal lobe origin. Nevertheless, its close association with localization-related epilepsies makes TIRDA an epileptogenic finding.

Sporadic temporal slowing, in contrast, does not have the same specificity of TIRDA in MTLE and is not epileptogenic. To maintain specificity of TIRDA compared to sporadic slowing, many conservatively reserve TIRDA for activity that truly appears only in rhythmic bursts and is recurrent during the recording.

Clinical Pearls

1. TIRDA is focal, intermittent, rhythmic delta activity that is potentially epileptogenic. It is the best documented epileptogenic finding that is not epileptiform.
2. TIRDA in suspected MTLE is highly predictive of side of seizure onset.

REFERENCES
1. Geyer JD, Bilir E, Faught E, et al: Significance of interictal temporal lobe delta activity for localization of the primary epileptogenic region. Neurology 1999; 52:202–205.
2. Normand MM, Wszolek ZK, Klass DW: Temporal intermittent rhythmic delta activity in electroencephalograms. J Clin Neurophysiol 1995; 12:280–284.

PATIENT 69

A 30-year-old man with complex partial seizures

An EEG is requested in a 30-year-old man who experienced an exacerbation of complex partial seizures despite documented anticonvulsant medication compliance. Medications are carbamazepine and phenytoin.

The patient is awake during the recording.

Question: What are the location and source of focal delta activity?

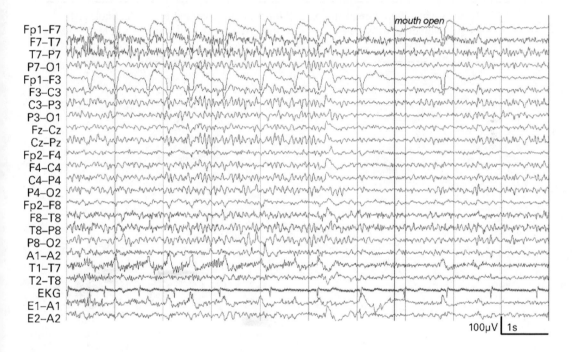

Answer: Frequent slow-wave discharges are present in the left frontotemporal channels. The source is left eye movement artifact in a subject with an enucleated right eye.

Discussion: Admittedly, the EEG technologist should document any usual physical features of the patient, such as skull defects and scars, or, as in this case, an enucleated eye.

Even in the absence of eye leads, eye movement artifact can usually be distinguished from frontal delta activity. Eye movement artifact is typically confined to the first two channels of a longitudinal montage, whereas most frontal delta activity of brain origin is broadly distributed.

Clinical Pearls

1. Physical characteristics of the patient must be documented by the technologist.
2. Eye movement artifact is usually confined to frontopolar and frontotemporal fields.

PATIENT 70

A 28-year-old woman with psychic auras

A 28-year-old woman presents with feelings of dissociation and déja vu that have been occurring for the previous 2 years. She is taking no medications.

The recording is made with the patient awake. The sample is shown in bipolar longitudinal and right-ear referential montages.

Question: What is the finding in the diagram?

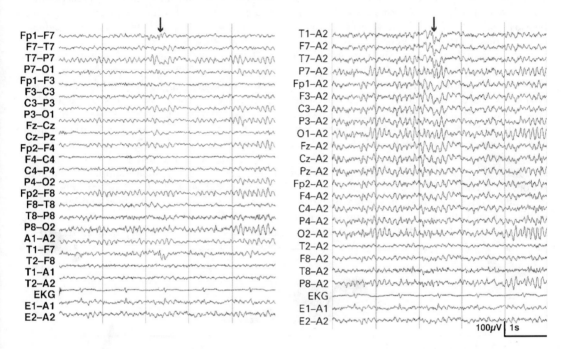

Answer: Left anterior midtemporal theta activity.

Discussion: Sporadic, subtle slowing is a recurrent problem in interpretation. In adults, slowing in the temporal regions is particularly vexing, and clinical significance varies with the type of slowing encountered and the age of the patient.

The most common of ambiguous slowings are brief bursts of low to medium amplitude (<50 μV) theta activities that occur synchronously bilaterally and often have a left-sided predominance. Retrospective studies demonstrate that this pattern may be an age-related phenomenon and occurs in elderly, asymptomatic individuals. These bursts of theta activity have been attributed to occult or symptomatic cerebrovascular disease.

One important confounder is the contribution of drowsiness. Bitemporally predominant, diffusely distributed bursts of theta activities frequently occur with onset of drowsy state. Many benign epileptiform transients also have a predilection for drowsiness and light sleep. Interpreters should review the record carefully for other evidence of drowsiness and should observe whether suspicious slowing is also present during the recording of full wakefulness.

Another confounder more prevalent with the use of digital EEG is the well-intended but overenthusiastic use of too-high sensitivity to increase the amplitude of records consisting of low-amplitude activities. Slowings that are not apparent at a common sensitivity of 7 μV/mm or its peak-to-peak equivalent should be greeted skeptically.

In comparison to theta activity, sporadic temporal delta activity in the waking adult record is usually abnormal and indicates localized neuronal dysfunction. Unfortunately, no prospective studies provide clear guidelines that specify how much asymmetry or frequency limits denote normal from abnormal for certain age groups. Nevertheless, older age, more symmetry and synchronicity, and more theta frequencies indicate insignificant slowings, whereas younger age, asymmetry, and more delta frequencies indicate significant slowings.

This patient's case shows significant theta slowing in the left anterior temporal region. It interrupts ongoing alpha rhythm (thus drowsiness is not present), it is clearly lateralized to the left, and it occurs in a relatively young patient.

The current case is also a good demonstration of the use of the A1-A2 channel used in the majority of examples in this book. Its relatively long interelectrode distance amplifies temporal activities and acts as a kind of semaphore that "flags" potential temporal abnormalities. Significance of findings, however, must be determined in context of the usual channels of the 10–20 bipolar montage.

Clinical Pearls

1. Temporal slowing must be interpreted with caution: Greater age, symmetry, and frequency suggest no clinical significance.

2. In viewing low-amplitude recordings, a too-high sensitivity may artificially inflate the relative importance of insignificant slowing.

3. An ear-ear (or temporal-temporal) channel included in bipolar montages is a helpful adjunct in the examination of potential temporal abnormalities.

PATIENT 71

A 6-year-old boy with bizarre behavior

A 6-year-old boy has recent episodes of bizarre behavior, such as wandering and violent outbursts. He is also being treated for attention-deficit disorder.

The recording is made with the patient awake. Medications include clonidine and Dexedrine.

Questions: What is the abnormality in photic driving responses? What is the background activity of the left hemisphere compared to the right?

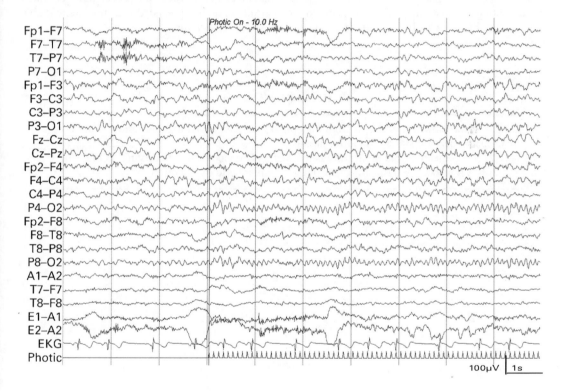

Answers: Photic driving response is asymmetric, appearing only at the right occipital region. The presence of left parasagittal theta activities during wakefulness, along with abnormal photic driving, suggests a physiologic abnormality of the left hemisphere.

Discussion: Although discrete lesions may cause the emergence of focal slowing, they may also cause alterations in normal activities or alterations in responses to activation procedures.

Asymmetry of photic driving suggests the presence of an ipsilateral physiologic or anatomic lesion. Although it rarely may be the sole abnormality, the lack of photic driving on one side usually occurs with other evidence of posterior or hemispheric dysfunction, as in this case. The corroborating evidence of left hemisphere dysfunction is diffusely distributed theta activities that are more predominant anteriorly and across the left hemisphere.

Neuroimaging with MRI failed to disclose any visible source of focal slowing and photic asymmetry in this case. A repeat recording disclosed left centroparietal spikes. With time, further observation confirmed suspicions that violent behaviors and wandering were postictal symptoms, and that brief staring spells with minimal automatisms—previously unappreciated complex partial seizures—preceded the more remarkable postictal symptoms.

Clinical Pearls

1. Focal slowing can result from nonepileptogenic or epileptogenic lesions that may not be present on standard neuroimaging.

2. Asymmetry of photic driving is marked by absence of photic driving on one side and is a nonspecific indicator of ipsilateral hemispheric dysfunction.

PATIENT 72

A 28-year-old woman with left intracranial hemorrhage

An EEG is requested to evaluate a 28-year-old woman with fluctuating mental status following a left thalamic hemorrhage. She is taking phenytoin, digoxin, and lisinopril.

The recording is made with the patient awake and slightly confused.

Question: How does the persistence and distribution of alpha rhythm differ between points *a* and *b?*

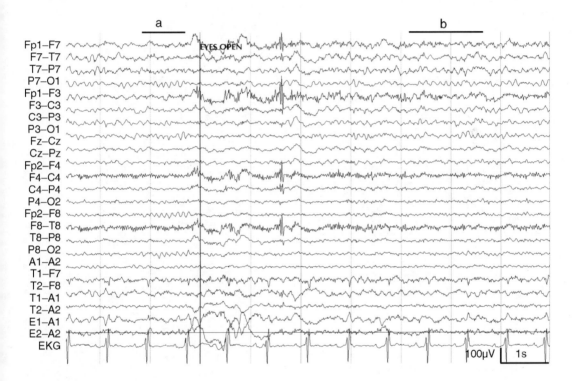

Answer: A brief run of posteriorly dominant, symmetric, low-amplitude ~9.5 cps alpha rhythm is present at point *a*. A slightly slower, ~8.5 cps posteriorly dominant rhythm is at point *b* that is unusual because it persists on the left side only, whereas it attenuates normally on the right side after eye opening.

Discussion: Focal lesions sometimes alter the characteristics of normal activities. *Bancaud's* phenomenon is the persistence of alpha rhythm after eye opening on one side, indicating ipsilateral hemispheric dysfunction.

REFERENCE

1. Bancaud J, Hecaen H, Lairy GC: Modifications de la reactivitie EEG, troubles de fonctions symboliques et troubles confusionnels dans les lesions hemispherics localisees. Electroencephalogr Clin Neurophysiol 1955; 7:295–302.

PATIENT 73

A 55-year-old woman with intractable epilepsy
after corticectomy

A 55-year-old woman undergoes epilepsy surgery to remove an epileptic focus near the somatosensory region of the right parietal cortex. The seizures consist of severe pain involving the left hand. Although seizures are successfully abolished by surgery, she has an independent seizure focus causing medically intractable complex partial seizures. Earlier intracranial monitoring confirms the origin of seizures within the right hippocampus. Neuroimaging findings and the symptoms of the seizure are consistent with right mesial temporal lobe epilepsy.

This sample is from an overnight video-EEG because of a spontaneous exacerbation in the frequency of seizures. The patient is taking carbamazepine and phenobarbital.

The patient is awake but sedated following administration of oral lorazepam.

Questions: What is the source of right central alpha activities? What are two other abnormalities in this sample?

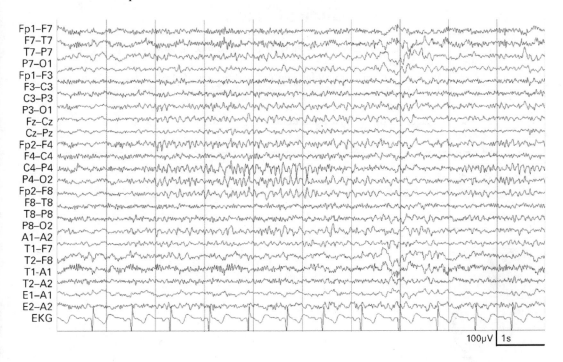

100μV | 1s

Answer: The source of right central alpha activities is breach rhythm (skull defect). Two abnormalities are enhancement of beta activities from medication effect and sporadic delta activities in the left anterior midtemporal region, indicating localized physiologic dysfunction.

Discussion: Breach rhythm denotes the distortion of activities resulting from abnormalities in underlying bone density. Historically, there are two variants.

The more specific type, pictured here, consists of medium-amplitude bursts of rhythmic, arciform, alpha frequency activities that resemble enhanced mu rhythm.

Less specifically, breach rhythm may refer to any focal enhancement of amplitude over skull defects, an enhancement that especially favors faster frequencies. Although some prefer the term *breach rhythm* to denote enhancement of the mu rhythm and *breach activities* to refer to any enhanced background activities, the overall effects of bony defects of cortical activity are the same.

The tissues that separate cortical activities from scalp electrodes not only attenuate the amplitude of electrical signal but also act as a high-frequency filter. The skull contributes the most to the overall impedance of the scalp EEG. Estimates of the impedances of the scalp are 1 kΩ, the skull 40 kΩ, and the dura mater 12 kΩ. Changes to the skull may be subtle; missing bone, as well as healed bone, can similarly alter scalp recordings.

To help in interpretation, the EEG technologist must provide a sketch or description of any abnormalities of the scalp.

Clinical Pearls

1. Breach rhythms result from underlying impedance changes resulting from abnormalities of the underlying skull.

2. Focal enhancement of amplitudes and overexpression of faster frequency activities from breach rhythms are not abnormalities in themselves but artifactual changes that must be taken into account during interpretation.

3. The EEG technologist must document any abnormalities of the scalp as part of the recording.

REFERENCES

1. Cobb WA, Guiloff RJ, Cast J: Breach rhythm: The EEG related to skull defects. Electroencephalogr Clin Neurophysiol 1979; 47:251–271.
2. Remond A: Origin transformation of electrical activities which result in the electroencephalogram. In Handbook of Electroencephalography and Clinical Neurophysiology. Amsterdam, Elsevier, 1977, p 21.

PATIENT 74

A 70-year-old man with altered mental state

A 70-year-old man presents after a burn injury with confusion and disorientation. He had undergone a coronary bypass several years before. Medications are albuterol, lisinopril, and digoxin. He is on no sedative medications during the tracing but received opiates for presumptive pain 2 hours before.

The patient is lethargic, intubated, and unable to follow commands.

Questions: What are the activities present at sample *a* compared to later in the recording at sample *b,* after the technologist applies mild painful stimulus? What do the changes imply regarding the patient's level of consciousness and etiology of confusion?

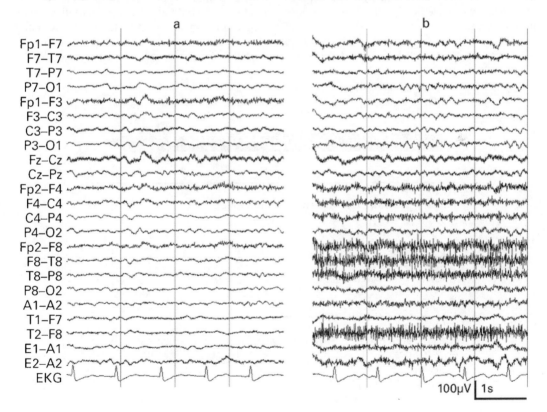

Answers: Predominantly low-amplitude, diffusely distributed delta activities during sample *a;* higher-amplitude, posteriorly dominant theta activities and muscle artifacts during sample *b,* after patient stimulation. Diffuse, reactive delta and theta activities are most consistent with moderate bihemispheric dysfunction on a toxic or metabolic basis.

Discussion: Encephalopathy is a general term denoting any alteration from normal consciousness. Traditionally, disorders of consciousness result from pathology affecting both cerebral hemispheres or the brainstem. The EEG is exquisitely sensitive in detecting encephalopathy because changes in the EEG correlate strongly with the severity of cerebral dysfunction. Because EEG can only record cortical activity, the EEG in cases of coma that do not involve the hemispheres, for example, locked-in syndrome and psychogenic coma, may be normal.

The table below outlines the spectrum of levels of consciousness and corresponding EEG patterns. Do not infer from the diagram that EEG findings march lock-step from one finding to another in sequence; indeed, not all patients show every corresponding EEG finding as they transition from drowsiness to lethargy to coma. Nevertheless, each finding pertaining to encephalopathy usually indicates similar levels of consciousness among patients.

Changes in EEG corresponding to severity of bihemispheric dysfunction can be described in terms of background frequency, amplitude, reactivity, and morphology.

Frequency. In general, a decline in level of consciousness corresponds to more slowing of the predominant frequency of the tracing. In lighter stages of encephalopathy, the alpha rhythm may slow in frequency. Progression may cause the alpha rhythm to be replaced altogether by theta or delta activity. The persistence of theta or delta activity increases with worsening consciousness, appearing in brief bursts in mild lethargy and in continuous runs in stupor.

Because background rhythms of the EEG arise from thalamocortical-corticothalamic reciprocal activity, diffuse slowing is evidence that ascending input to the thalamus is affected or that axonal connections between thalamus and cortex are disrupted or impaired.

Amplitude. During mild encephalopathies, the overall amplitude of activity may increase, reflective of normal waking activities being replaced by predominant theta or delta activities. However, as neuronal dysfunction worsens, the number of neurons able to contribute to EEG

level of consciousness:

alert awake	drowsy	lethargic	stuporous	comatose	brain dead

worse encephalopathy →

frequency:

alpha rhythm	slowing loss alpha	intermittent slowing	continuous slowing
		theta	delta

amplitude:

normal	increased		suppressed	electro–cerebral silence

morphology:

	enhanced beta	triphasic waves PEDS/PLEDS	suppression burst	alpha/theta coma

reactivity:

reactive	paradoxical reactivity		unreactive	

Effects of Diffuse Encephalopathy on EEG

activity decreases. Suppression, therefore, corresponds to severe encephalopathy in which underlying neurons have become inactive or are lost. The loss of all cerebral activity is termed *electrocerebral silence* (ECS) and is one of the criteria of brain death.

Morphology. Certain patterns of waveforms appear during bihemispheric encephalopathy. Some patterns correspond closely with certain states of consciousness, such as IRDA or triphasic waves that appear in lethargic patients. Alpha coma, or unreactive, diffuse alpha activity, corresponds to severe coma, as do bursts of high-amplitude activities separated by periods of suppression (suppression-burst). Some patterns are associated with specific etiologies of encephalopathy. *Periodic epileptiform discharges* (PEDs) are associated with spongiform encephalopathies, such as Jakob-Creutzfeldt disease. Ictal discharges in the form of rhythmic or periodic discharges may be present in patients with *nonconvulsive status epilepticus* (NCSE).

Reactivity. Loss of endogenously mediated changes in activity states and absence of responses to environmental stimuli indicate worse bihemispheric dysfunction. Stimuli ranging from verbal questioning to mild shaking to painful stimuli should be used to provoke changes in clinical state and EEG findings. All EEGs should contain a portion during which arousal is present spontaneously or induced by the technologist.

Although the EEG is highly sensitive in reflecting level of consciousness, in most cases, it is also nonspecific. Many different etiologies of diffuse encephalopathy can cause the same EEG finding.

In this patient's case, background activities of mixed theta and delta range activities are reactive. No ongoing seizure activity is present. Therefore, the most likely cause of the patient's waxing and waning disorientation is mild to moderate bihemispheric dysfunction on a toxic or metabolic basis. The patient's mental status is thought to be multifactorial in etiology.

Clinical Pearls

1. Findings in EEG in bihemispheric dysfunction are highly sensitive but poorly specific.

2. Worsening encephalopathy correlates with slowing of background frequencies, suppression of amplitude, and loss of reactivity.

REFERENCE

1. Plum F, Posner JB: Pathologic physiology of signs and symptoms of coma. In Plum F, Posner JB (eds): The Diagnosis of Stupor and Coma, 3rd ed.. Philadelphia, F.A. Davis, 1982, pp 1–86.

PATIENT 75

A 51-year-old woman with confusion after electroconvulsive therapy

A 51-year-old woman has persistent but variable confusion following electroconvulsive therapy for major depression. The neurology consultant is concerned about possible nonconvulsive status epilepticus. Medications are venlafaxine and trazodone.

The tracing is recorded with the patient awake but confused.

Question: How are the posterior rhythms evident at *a* and *c* unusual in relationship to findings at *b?*

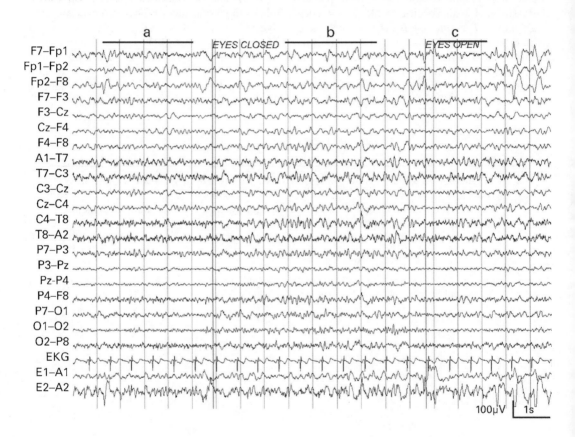

Effects of Diffuse Encephalopathy on EEG

Answer: 7–7.5 cps posteriorly dominant activities persist during eye opening (a) and are replaced by slower-frequency activities after eye closure (b). Alpha rhythm paradoxically recurs after eye opening (c). Paradoxical alpha rhythm indicates mild encephalopathy.

Discussion: Just as alpha rhythm may slow in cases of mild encephalopathy, the alpha rhythm may manifest abnormal reactivity as well. In this case, an alpha rhythm—albeit one abnormally slow—persists during eye opening rather than eye closure. *Paradoxical alpha rhythm* emerges during mild encephalopathy. The arousal elicited by brief eye opening may cause emergence of an organized posterior rhythm that would be otherwise absent in the baseline, pathologically lethargic state.

In this patient's case, the appearance of paradoxical alpha rhythm correlates with other findings of slow alpha rhythm during periods of maximum arousal. Ongoing electrographic seizure activity is not present; therefore, her current state is not due to nonconvulsive status epilepticus. There are case reports of NCSE arising after electroconvulsive therapy, but these are exceptional and rare. Therefore, her EEG supports a conclusion that encephalopathy is the result of metabolic or toxic bihemispheric dysfunction, or remains as a direct effect of electroconvulsive therapy, a broad diagnosis that requires clinical clarification from her primary physicians.

Clinical Pearls

1. Paradoxical alpha rhythm is the emergence of an occipital alpha rhythm after eye opening. It indicates deficient arousal or mild encephalopathy.

2. Changes in normal rhythms can indicate abnormality. Alpha rhythm must be interpreted in the correct context of patient arousal and reactivity.

REFERENCE

1. Varma NK, Lee SI: Nonconvulsive status epilepticus following electroconvulsive therapy. Neurology 1992; 42(1):263–264.

PATIENT 76

A 77-year-old woman with depression and parkinsonism

A 77-year-old woman with idiopathic Parkinson's disease is about to be treated for intractable depression with electroconvulsive therapy. An EEG is requested to help evaluate for encephalopathy. Medications are not listed.

The sample seen in a referential montage is recorded with the patient awake. The technologist noted intermittent parkinsonian tremor. Normal alpha rhythm is seen in an earlier portion of the recording.

Question: Does the sample provide evidence of cerebral dysfunction?

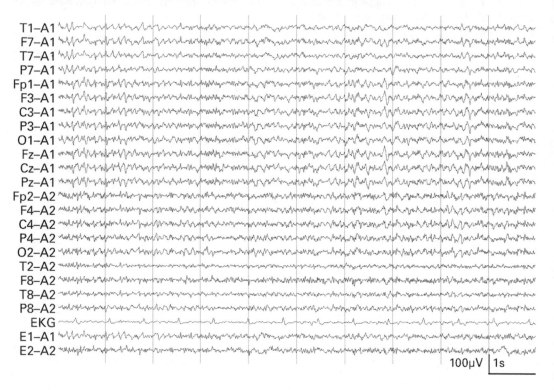

Answer: The tracing shows rhythmic ~6 cps theta activities that are broadly distributed but are more evident across the left hemisphere. Faster activities in the alpha and beta frequency bands are visible intermittently. The resting tremor in Parkinson's disease has a frequency of ~6 Hz. Artifact, not encephalopathy, is the source of slowing of waking activities in this sample.

Discussion: The interpreter is often dependent upon the technologist to provide information to aid in interpretation. In this case, three findings help in the diagnosis of artifact:

1. The distribution of theta activity is unusual for mild encephalopathy; slowing of the posterior rhythm is more common, and this sample lacks any evidence of a posterior dominance of theta activity.

2. The technologist's notation of intermittent tremor, combined with the knowledge that the common frequency of Parkinsonian tremor is 5–6 Hz, should make the interpreter suspicious of the source of the signal.

3. Referential montages, because of increased interelectrode distance, are more susceptible to obscuration from movement artifact than bipolar montages.

The technologist could have elected to place a hand movement monitor to confirm the source of the signal. Current digital EEG systems commonly offer simultaneous video, so that direct observation of the patient can also disclose the source of artifact.

Clinical Pearls

1. Movement artifact may obscure cerebral activities. Careful notation by EEG technologists and healthy skepticism of the EEG reader are required for proper interpretation.

2. Referential montages are more susceptible to obscuration from movement artifact because of increased interelectrode distances and use of a common reference.

PATIENT 77

A 59-year-old diabetic woman with lethargy

A 59-year-old diabetic woman has three syncope-like episodes. It is determined that she misdosed an oral hypoglycemic agent and had transient hypoglycemia. She remains obtunded despite correction of blood glucose. Other medications are ACE inhibitors and warfarin.

This EEG is obtained during confused wakefulness.

Question: What is the pattern *(bar)* and its interpretation?

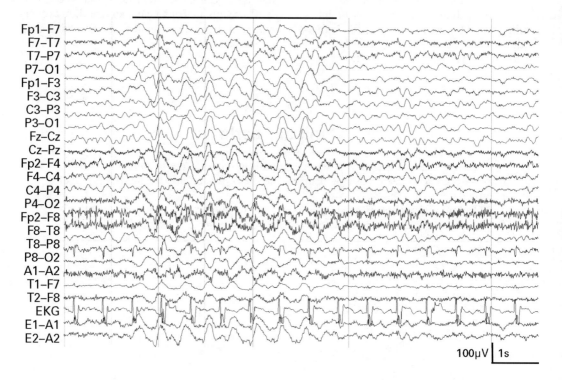

Effects of Diffuse Encephalopathy on EEG

Answer: *Frontally dominant intermittent rhythmic delta activity* (FIRDA) indicates a mild-to-moderate encephalopathy of toxic or metabolic origin.

Discussion: FIRDA consists of rhythmic, 2-cps medium- to high-amplitude delta activities. Delta activities are generalized but appear with highest amplitudes in anterior head regions. Bursts of rhythmic delta activity typically last 2–5 seconds. Waveforms have a sinusoidal or sawtooth morphology. Patient stimulation and spontaneous arousal can decrease persistence of FIRDA.

FIRDA usually corresponds to a state of lethargy or mild-to-moderate encephalopathy during which arousal is possible but a normal level of consciousness is not obtained. Correspondingly, alpha rhythm is frequently absent in patients with FIRDA, which most often appears during background activities of poorly organized theta activities.

FIRDA indicates that a toxic or metabolic cause of encephalopathy is present. Historically, FIRDA was thought to represent "projected rhythms" from deep, midline lesions, especially those that were associated with increased intracranial pressure. Indeed, some authorities note that if FIRDA occurs during wakefulness or during normal waking EEG activity, it suggests intrinsic brain disease, whereas FIRDA accompanied by slowing of background activities during lethargy is toxic-metabolic in origin.

Clinical Pearl

FIRDA is usually evidence of mild-to-moderate encephalopathies of toxic or metabolic origin.

REFERENCE
1. Zurek R, Schiemann Delgado J, Froescher W, Niedermeyer E: Frontal intermittent rhythmical delta activity and anterior bradyrhythmia. Clin Electroencephalogr 1985; 16:1–10.

PATIENT 78

A 79-year-old woman with spells

A 79-year-old woman with epilepsy is evaluated for spells that continue even after increasing the dosage of phenytoin. Other medications are aspirin and hydrochlorothiazide.

The tracing is recorded with the patient awake.

Question: Does the tracing provide evidence of cerebral dysfunction?

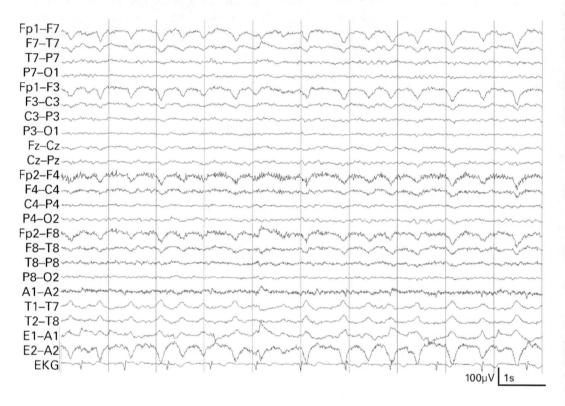

Effects of Diffuse Encephalopathy on EEG

Answer: The tracing shows rhythmic 2 cps delta activity in the anterior channels. Phase reversals in EOG channels reveal that rhythmic activity stems from rhythmic eye movement. Low-amplitude alpha activities are also present.

Discussion: EOG distinguishes eye movement artifact from cerebral anterior delta activity or FIRDA. In this patient's case, the waking EEG is otherwise normal.

Clinical Pearls

1. Eye movement will cause phase-reversing potentials in EOG channels.
2. Eye movements may be mistaken for cerebral anterior delta activity.

PATIENT 79

A 55-year-old man with psychosis

A 55-year-old man presents with psychosis, and EEG is requested to evaluate organic causes of delirium.

The tracing is recorded with the patient awake on no medications.

Questions: What are the sources of signal at point *a* and point *b?* Are these FIRDA?

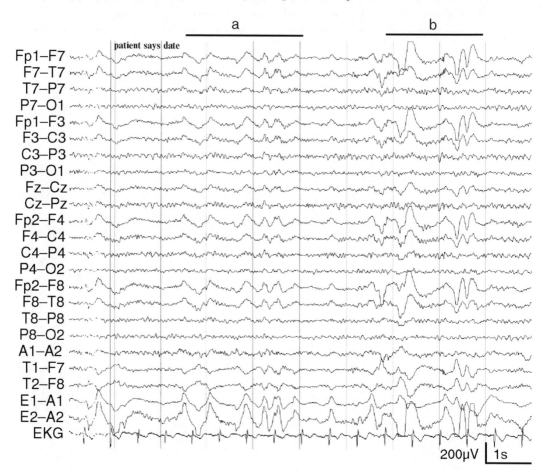

Effects of Diffuse Encephalopathy on EEG

Answers: The source of signal at point *a* is glossokinetic artifact during talking, which causes the frontally dominant artifact that is in-phase in EOG channels and is higher in amplitude in EOG than in frontal channels. The source of signal at point *b* is eye movement artifact, which causes the frontally dominant artifact that is out-of-phase in EOG channels.

Discussion: EOG is helpful in distinguishing eye movement artifact from other sources of anterior slowing.

Eye movement causes potentials that phase-reverse in EOG channels. Activity from sources other than eyes causes potentials that are in-phase.

Tongue movement (glossokinetic artifact) produces artifact that is in-phase in EOG channels. The tongue is closer to EOG electrodes than cerebral electrodes. Therefore, artifacts from the tongue will be higher in potential in EOG than in cerebral channels, if the sensitivities are set to the same level.

Cerebral activity remains in-phase in eye lead channels.

In this patient's case, the ability to distinguish artifact from cerebral slowing helps determine that the patient's symptoms are more likely psychiatric than organic in origin.

Clinical Pearls

1. Eye movement causes frontally dominant artifact that phase-reverses in EOG channels.

2. Tongue movement causes frontally dominant artifact that is larger in potential in EOG channels than in cerebral channels and does not phase-reverse in EOG channels.

3. Frontal slowing of cerebral origin does not phase-reverse in eye lead channels and is higher in potential in cerebral channels than in eye lead channels.

PATIENT 80

A 49-year-old woman with pseudotumor cerebri and intermittent lethargy

A 49-year-old woman has pseudotumor cerebri. Spells of inattention or lethargy are observed. There is a question of absence seizures. Intracranial pressure, determined by lumbar puncture, is found to be elevated. Medications are acetazolamide and an unnamed antihypertensive medication. This EEG is obtained during wakefulness.

Questions: What is the predominant finding in the first half of the sample *(bar a)*? In the second half of the sample *(bar b)*?

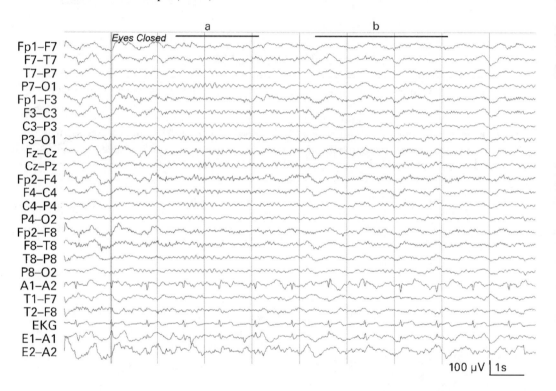

Effects of Diffuse Encephalopathy on EEG

Answers: A normal alpha rhythm of ~10 cps is present during the first portion of the recording. FIRDA occurs during the second.

Discussion: FIRDA usually occurs on slowed, disorganized background activities of wakefulness and, in that setting, indicates a toxic-metabolic etiology of encephalopathy.

Occasionally, FIRDA occurs on otherwise normal activities of wakefulness. Not all authorities agree on the specificity of FIRDA in this situation. Some studies show that intrinsic brain disease, especially deep-seated midline lesions, or lesions causing increased intracranial pressure, are associated with FIRDA. In this patient's case, FIRDA appears to correlate with high intracranial pressure, but FIRDA should not be considered a diagnostic finding or a screening test for intracranial pressure problems, such as pseudotumor cerebri.

FIRDA may appear in other situations in an otherwise normal EEG:

1. FIRDA may appear briefly during drowsiness in adults.

2. FIRDA may appear as "build-up" phenomena during hyperventilation.

3. In neonatal studies, intermittent runs of anteriorly dominant delta activities may briefly appear. Such "anterior dysrhythmia" has no clear pathologic basis.

Clinical Pearls

1. FIRDA, in the setting of normal activities of wakefulness, can occur in intrinsic brain disease, especially in the setting of increased intracranial pressure.

2. Anteriorly dominant rhythmic delta activity, limited to hyperventilation or to drowsiness, may occur in normal individuals.

REFERENCES

1. Fariello RG, Orrison W, Blanco G, Reyes PF: Neuroradiological correlates of frontally predominant intermittent rhythmic delta activity (FIRDA). Electroencephalogr Clin Neurophysiol 1982; 54(2):194–202.
2. Zurek R, Schiemann Delgado J, Froescher W, Niedermeyer E: Frontal intermittent rhythmical delta activity and anterior bradyrhythmia. Clin Electroencephalogr 1985; 16:1–10.

PATIENT 81

A 5-year-old girl with lethargy

A 5-year-old girl presents with persistent lethargy following a new-onset generalized tonic clonic seizure that occurs about 24 hours before the tracing.

The recording is performed with the patient aroused but confused. She is on no medications.

Questions: What is the predominant rhythmic activity *(bar)?* Is background activity normal for awake state?

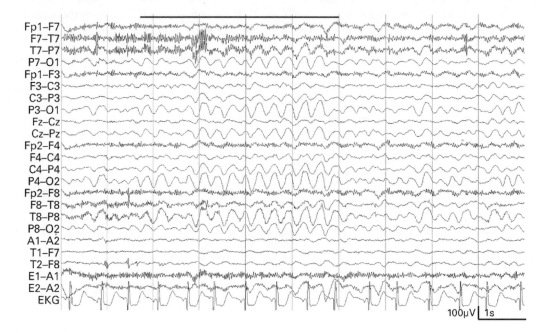

Effects of Diffuse Encephalopathy on EEG

Answers: *Occipitally dominant intermittent rhythmic delta activity* (OIRDA) is especially prominent under the bar. Background activities are too slow for age and state. The findings indicate an encephalopathy of toxic, metabolic, or postictal origin.

Discussion: OIRDA has the same electroencephalographic features as FIRDA, but delta activities appear with highest amplitudes in posterior head regions.

OIRDA is traditionally the pediatric equivalent to FIRDA, corresponding to a state of lethargy and indicative of mild-to-moderate encephalopathy. The posterior, rather than anterior, predominance of rhythmic slowing in children is attributed to the caudal-to-rostral pattern of myelination in the maturing brain.

OIRDA, however, is seen in a wider variety of diseases that do not involve encephalopathy.

Most importantly, OIRDA is a frequent finding in childhood absence epilepsy and may be seen in other, generalized epilepsies. In other words, OIRDA may be epileptogenic, a finding analogous to TIRDA and temporal lobe epilepsies. OIRDA, when seen in patients with absence epilepsy, is considered by some authorities as an indicator that absence seizures will not spontaneously remit or may later evolve to generalized motor seizures.

Similar to FIRDA, OIRDA may also indicate deep, midline lesions that affect intracranial pressure.

In this patient's case, background slowing of waking activities could be attributed to postictal or other encephalopathies, and OIRDA could be an epileptogenic finding. Another possibility is that both background slowing and OIRDA merely indicate encephalopathy. Repeat recording will be required to help differentiate between the two possibilities.

Clinical Pearls

1. OIRDA, especially in the presence of disorganized, slow background activities, is a nonspecific marker of mild-to-moderate toxic-metabolic encephalopathies in children.

2. OIRDA carries a high association with childhood absence epilepsy and other idiopathic generalized epilepsies.

REFERENCE

1. Gullipalli D, Fountain NB: Clinical correlation of occipital intermittent rhythmic delta activity. J Clin Neurophysiol 2003; 20:35–41.

PATIENT 82

An 85-year-old woman with stupor and jaundice

An 85-year-old woman presents with jaundice and stupor. No medical history is available. She is treated with charcoal lavage and lactulose.

The EEG is recorded at bedside with the patient poorly responsive. No CNS-active medications are present.

Questions: What is the morphology of the rhythmic discharges? What features of these waveforms suggest a toxic-metabolic origin of the patient's stupor?

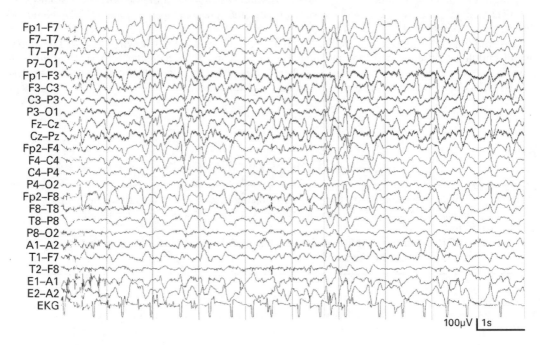

Effects of Diffuse Encephalopathy on EEG

Answers: Rhythmic waveforms have a triphasic morphology. Rhythmic triphasic waves that are generalized and appear on the scalp with a lag between anterior and posterior regions are seen in toxic-metabolic causes of stupor.

Discussion: *Triphasic waves* typically appear in rhythmic trains at a frequency of 2 cps or slightly slower. They are generalized and usually anteriorly dominant. Most triphasic waves are symmetric across the hemispheres, but some side-to-side differences in amplitude or persistence can occur, as seen in the current case of hepatic encephalopathy.

The morphologies of triphasic waves may vary considerably by montage but characteristically assume a ''dog-leg'' shape. A finding helpful in the identification of triphasic waves is that the major component of the triphasic wave often demonstrates a lag in timing between anterior and posterior regions. Anterior-to-posterior *phase lags* are rarely more prolonged than 125 msec but are present in the majority of triphasic waves of toxic-metabolic origin. Longitudinal bipolar montages exaggerate phase lag, and referential montages minimize it. A helpful technique to

check for phase lag is to use fast paper speed to allow close examination of the timing of the major components of triphasic waves in adjacent channels.

Triphasic waves were first studied in the setting of hepatic encephalopathy, and are certainly highly associated with hepatic dysfunction. When triphasic waves, stupor, and hepatic failure are seen together, mortality is high. However, triphasic waves are neither specific nor sensitive in determining the exact cause of a coma. The pattern may appear in various encephalopathies of toxic or metabolic origin.

Triphasic waves, however, are, in some reports, specific for a certain level of consciousness, a ''twilight state'' between lethargy and frank stupor. Some care must be made to distinguish rhythmic triphasic waves from spike and slow-wave complexes indicative of status epilepticus.

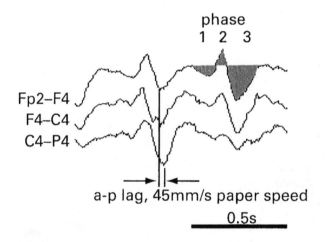

Clinical Pearls

1. Triphasic waves consist of rhythmic, 2-cps, generalized, anteriorly dominant triphasic discharges.

2. The common anterior-to-posterior phase lag of the major component of triphasic waves can be accentuated by longitudinal bipolar montages at fast paper speeds.

3. Triphasic waves may be seen in patients with states between lethargy and stupor and indicate a toxic-metabolic origin of encephalopathy.

Effects of Diffuse Encephalopathy on EEG

REFERENCES

1. Bickford RG, Butt HR: Hepatic coma: The electroencephalographic pattern. J Clin Invest 1955; 34:790–799.
2. Fisch BJ, Klass DW: The diagnostic specificity of triphasic wave patterns. Electroencephalogr Clin Neurophysiol 1988; 70:1–8.

PATIENT 83

A 61-year-old man with postoperative confusion

An EEG is requested in a 61-year-old man who remains stuporous following resection of colon cancer. He is on no CNS-active medications beyond general anesthesia 12 hours before. He is intubated.

Question: Does the patient's encephalopathy arise from intraoperative anoxia, persistent anesthesia, or other causes of toxic-metabolic encephalopathy?

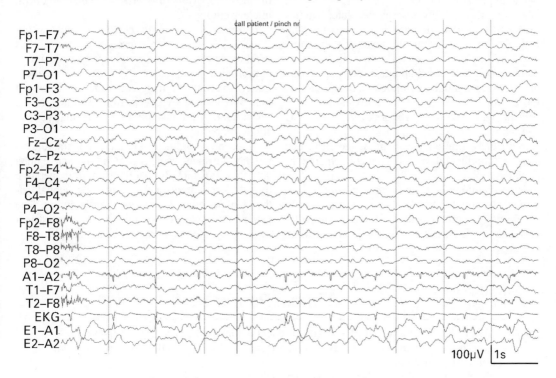

Answer: The sample contains unreactive arrhythmic generalized delta activities. Although the pattern is consistent with severe encephalopathies, it does not indicate the cause of encephalopathy.

Discussion: An EEG composed of generalized, arrhythmic delta activity that is unreactive to external stimulation indicates severe encephalopathy.

Early work was attempted to grade EEG findings to provide prognosis in stupor and coma. A traditional scheme is division of coma into four grades. Grades I and II correspond to reactive patterns, and grades III and IV to unreactive patterns ranging from arrhythmic delta activities, burst-suppression, and ECS.

However, with few exceptions, later studies disclosed that EEG findings in diffuse encephalopathies are sensitive to the level of consciousness but are neither specific for etiology nor predictive of outcome. Patients affected with disorders with potentially reversible courses, such as those from severe sedative intoxication, may present with profound abnormalities on EEG and recover.

With these limitations in mind, the EEG can answer important questions in the encephalopathic patient.

Is encephalopathy from certain etiologic categories? Although EEG findings are nonspecific for etiology, certain causes of encephalopathy have recurrent, classic findings. Metabolic-toxic causes commonly produce reactive diffuse slowing or specific patterns, such as triphasic waves. Periodic epileptiform discharges are associated with acute destructive lesions. Normal-appearing tracings can be seen in brainstem lesions.

Is encephalopathy caused by ongoing seizure activity? A greater appreciation of "subclinical status epilepticus" or nonconvulsive status epilepticus has lead to the increasing use of emergent EEG or prolonged bedside EEG in the acute or subacute evaluation of stupor or coma with unclear etiology.

Is prognosis grim in certain clinical situations? EEG, in certain causes of coma, such as cerebral hypoxia, can provide prognostic information that complements clinical examination. Patterns recorded during coma are not fixed but may fluctuate or evolve in time. In these cases, serial tracings are usually more informative than single recordings.

A second recording of this patient on the following day shows the same pattern of unreactive delta activities. It is thought that transient intraoperative hypoxia accounted for the patient's encephalopathy, but no other evidence is forthcoming. The patient is extubated but remains in a persistent vegetative state before discharge to hospice.

Clinical Pearls

1. An EEG correlates with severity of encephalopathy but usually not its etiology.
2. The prognostic value of EEG in coma is most helpful when the etiology is known or at least suspected.
3. Serial recordings offer improved specificity in prognostication.

REFERENCE

1. Synek VM: Prognostically important EEG coma patterns in diffuse anoxic and traumatic encephalopathies in adults. J Clin Neurophysiol 1988; 5:161–174.

PATIENT 84

A 71-year-old woman in stupor

An EEG is requested to determine etiology of spells of apnea and right upper-extremity posturing. The 71-year-old woman has an acute left hemisphere stroke and right hemisphere intracranial hemorrhage and undergoes surgical evacuation of the clot. She has a history of unspecified seizures.

The recording is performed with the patient stuporous. Medications are phenytoin and dexamethasone.

Question: What are the three abnormalities and two artifacts on this recording?

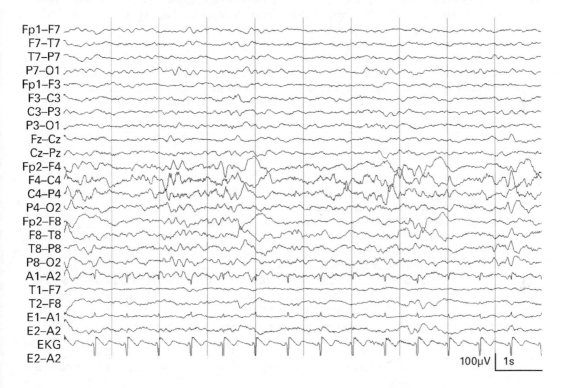

Answer: The three abnormalities are (1) background activities of diffuse, unreactive theta and delta activities; (2) focal arrhythmic delta activity across the right centroparietal region; and (3) right centroparietal spikes. The two artifacts are (1) right central enhanced beta activities and amplitudes consistent with breach rhythms and (2) EKG artifact in channels A1-A2 and E1-A1.

Discussion: Breach rhythms are focal changes arising from underlying conductive properties of the skull rather than from intrinsic brain abnormalities. The skull and overlying soft tissues act as both a high-frequency filter and as a sensitivity adjustment; the combination causes loss of amplitudes for all frequencies with a disproportionate loss of fast frequencies. Loss of skull, or even changes in bone thickness from healing surgery, reverse these effects and cause focal enhancement of fast frequencies.

Not only do fast frequencies in channels that overlie a skull breach appear out of proportion to those in uninvolved channels, but also the wider "frequency response" allows many waveforms to gain an epileptiform morphology. In comparison to clinically significant IEDs, artifactually enhanced "sharp" frequencies appear sharp only over the breach; IEDs, on the other hand, often have a potential field within and without the breach. Slow afterpotentials and other morphologic features, as discussed earlier, may aid in the separation of artifact from IEDs. In this case, spikes appear independently in central and parietal regions, and central spikes have a field that extends beyond the breach into the right parietal region.

Focal arrhythmic delta activities are also enhanced in amplitude, but the potential field of arrhythmic delta activity extends beyond the breach and indicates localized structural or physiologic dysfunction.

Finally, the background of this tracing consists of unreactive mixed theta and delta activities. This finding usually corresponds to clinical stupor in which arousal is minimal or pathologic.

Clinical Pearls

1. Breach rhythms consist of focally enhanced amplitudes of predominantly fast frequencies and arise from focal abnormalities of skull density.

2. Abnormalities underlying breach areas, such as focal arrhythmic delta activity or spike discharges, require typical morphologies and potential fields that project beyond the breach region to be accurately interpreted.

3. Diffuse, unreactive mixed delta and theta activities correspond to clinical states of stupor but are nonspecific consequences of severe metabolic-toxic disorders or from moderately severe diffuse structural abnormalities.

REFERENCE

1. Cobb WA, Guiloff RJ, Cast J: Breach rhythm: The EEG related to skull defects. Electroencephalogr Clin Neurophysiol 1979; 47:251–271.

PATIENT 85

A 16-year-old girl after motor vehicle accident and head trauma

A 16-year-old girl presents with episodes of leftward eye deviation following an unrestrained motor vehicle accident, closed head injury, multiple limb fractures, and subsequent waxing and waning stupor. Neuroimaging disclosed no intra-axial hemorrhages.

The technologist notes severe left-sided scalp edema but is able to place all electrodes to the 10–20 standard. Among various antibiotics and GI medications, the patient receives lorazepam, 2 mg 2 hours before the recording. The recording is performed in the surgical intensive care unit with the patient mildly sedated, confused, and poorly cooperative.

Question: Which hemisphere is worse?

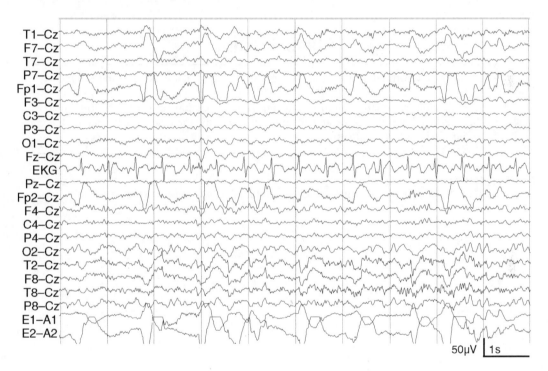

Answer: Neither, perhaps. The right temporal region shows medium-amplitude 6–7 cps theta activities that do not react to spontaneous eye opening or closure. Activities across the remainder of the scalp appear suppressed in amplitude. This suppression does not arise from intrinsic cerebral signals but is the result of attenuation of signal from scalp edema.

Discussion: Whereas localized lesions of the white matter generate focal slowing, lesions of the cortex tend to cause focal attenuation. Problematic, however, is that the amplitudes of potentials recorded from the scalp depend not only on neuronal populations but also upon the conductive properties of the intervening tissues and scalp electrodes.

Fluid collections, such as subdural hematomas, subdural hygromas, or epidural hematomas, can all attenuate signal by increasing the distance between cortex and electrodes. Similarly, severe scalp edema may increase recording distances in addition to altering the inherent impedance. Conversely, electrodes over regions of decreased distance and altered skull, such as after craniotomy for decompression, may record higher-than-normal amplitudes.

Clinical Pearls

1. Localized cortical lesions that cause focal loss of neurons may induce focal suppression.

2. Artifactual attenuation from underlying fluid collections or other abnormalities of the interface between cortex and scalp electrodes may attenuate signal, leaving the false impression of cortical suppression.

REFERENCE

1. Gloor P, Ball G, Schaul N: Brain lesions that produce delta waves in the EEG. Neurology 1977; 27:326–333.

PATIENT 86

A 34-year-old woman in a coma after cardiac arrest

A 34-year-old woman with congenital heart disease is comatose following cardiac arrest. An EEG is requested to evaluate possible seizures after repetitive jerks are observed. Prognosis is also requested.

The recording is made at bedside with the patient comatose and intubated. Some reactivity (emergence of theta activities) is noted at one point of the recording, and no motor seizure activity is observed. The montage is referenced to averaged ear inputs (AVG).

Question: What findings relevant to prognosis are seen in this EEG?

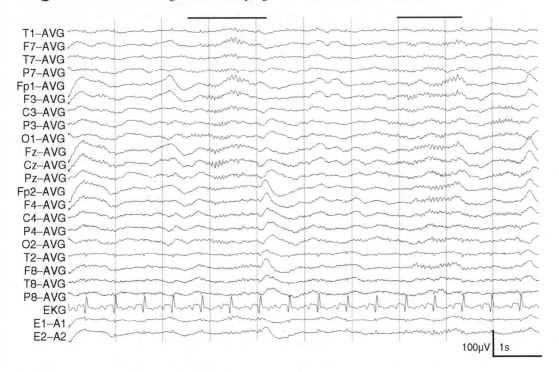

Answer: Bursts of centrally dominant 13-cps activities with a spindle-form morphology *(under bars)* are consistent with sleep spindles during a coma. Spindle coma is a pattern suggestive of favorable prognosis.

Discussion: Spindle coma refers to recordings of comatose patients in which bursts of beta activities resembling sleep spindles occur. The pattern in this case is consistent with sleep spindles: synchronous, bicentral, spindle-form bursts of alpha or low beta frequency activities.

The prognostic value of spindles during a coma is controversial. One problem is the basic limitation of EEG in the examination of encephalopathy: Patterns on EEG are not specific to etiology but to level of consciousness, and clinical outcome is usually determined by the underlying etiology. Comparison of the many studies that examine "spindle coma," therefore, is difficult because of differences in etiologies and patient selection. Nevertheless, some common features stand out.

First, in studies of patients with similar etiology of coma (historically head trauma), recurring spindles correlate with shorter durations of coma.

In longer, overnight recordings of comatose patients, the presence of spindles or other patterns of sleep implies intact sleep regulatory pathways and is linked with better outcomes than recordings that lack sleep patterns.

Second, in EEGs that include various causes of coma, spindle coma usually has no clear prognostic usefulness.

Third, in patients whose primary etiology of coma predicts grim prognosis, the presence of spindles does not clearly predict otherwise.

In this particular case of anoxic injury, care must be made to distinguish the alpha activity of spindles from the unreactive, monomorphic appearance of alpha activities in so-called "alpha coma," a pattern of poor prognosis in cerebral anoxia. The spindle-form nature of alpha activity and the reactivity of background activities distinguish this tracing from the more grim finding of alpha coma.

Clinical Pearls

1. The finding of sleep patterns—sleep spindles—in the EEG of a comatose patient is called *spindle coma*.

2. Spindle coma has historically been studied in traumatic brain injury, but it is not limited to that particular etiology.

3. Spindle coma, in highly selected and homogeneous patient groups, implies intact sleep regulatory pathways and is an indicator of relatively good prognosis in terms of avoidance of persistent vegetative state or death.

REFERENCES

1. Hansotia P, Gottschalk P, Green P, Zais D: Spindle coma: Incidence, clinicopathologic correlates, and prognostic value. Neurology 1981; 31:83–87.
2. Rumpl E, Prugger M, Bauer G, et al: Incidence and prognostic value of spindles in post-traumatic coma. Electroencephalogr Clin Neurophysiol 1983; 56:420–429.
3. Valente M, Placidi F, Oliveira AJ, et al: Sleep organization pattern as a prognostic marker at the subacute stage of post-traumatic coma. Clin Neurophysiol 2002; 113:1789–1805.

PATIENT 87

A 75-year-old man after aortic aneurysm dissection

A 75-year-old man presents in a coma after thoracic aortic artery dissection.
The recording is made at bedside with the patient intubated and unresponsive.

Question: What is this pattern seen in a coma?

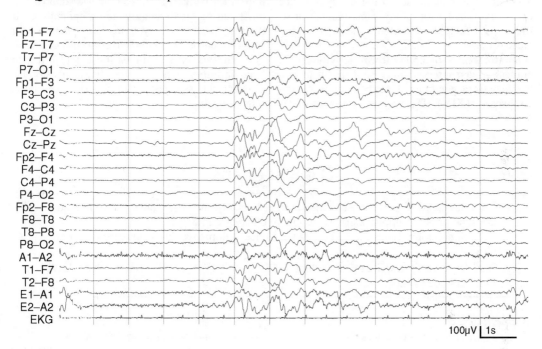

100µV | 1s

Answer: Suppression-burst.

Discussion: Suppression-burst consists of low-amplitude ($\sim$ <10 µV) background activity that is interrupted by quasi-periodic bursts of generalized, higher-amplitude, mixed-frequency activities. The morphology of bursts usually consists of disordered, mixed-frequency activities that last for 1–5 seconds. Interburst intervals typically range from 2–10 seconds. Increasing interburst intervals correspond to worsening states. Some designate the pattern according to persistence (suppression-burst for more suppression, burst-suppression for more frequent bursts), but either order is correct.

Shorter bursts of epileptiform activities with brief interburst intervals may be difficult to distinguish from generalized periodic epileptiform discharges (PEDs). The epileptiform discharges in PEDs, however, usually consist of broadly based, biphasic or polyphasic sharp discharges. PEDs, in addition, usually occur on background activities other than suppression; they interrupt ongoing activities rather than appear as the sole activity.

As discussed before, the prognosis of suppression-burst depends on the etiology. Anesthesia can induce suppression-burst; thiopental or propofol may be used at doses to cause suppression-burst during treatment of status epilepticus. In the case of cerebral hypoxia, most patients with suppression-burst fail to recover meaningful function. In this case, suppression-burst following hypoxic injury after prolonged hypoperfusion has a significant association with persistent vegetative state or death.

Clinical Pearls

1. Suppression-burst consists of recurrent bursts of mixed-frequency activities that are superimposed upon otherwise suppressed background.

2. Suppression-burst indicates a severe encephalopathy but is nonspecific to etiology.

3. In the setting of hypoxic coma, suppression-burst suggests lack of meaningful functional recovery.

REFERENCES
1. Gloor P, Ball G, Schaul N: Brain lesions that produce delta waves in the EEG. Neurology 1977; 27:326–333.
2. Synek VM: Prognostically important EEG coma patterns in diffuse anoxic and traumatic encephalopathies in adults. J Clin Neurophysiol 1988; 5:161–174.

Effects of Diffuse Encephalopathy on EEG

PATIENT 88

A 68-year-old man after cardiac arrest and coma

A 68-year-old man presents with a coma and occasional posturing and myoclonic jerks following cardiac arrest. There are no CNS-active medications. The patient is treated with a bolus of intravenous midazolam for presumptive seizure but is off all CNS-active medications for at least 12 hours.

The recording is performed at bedside with the intubated patient unresponsive to external stimulation.

Questions: How do the alpha activities here differ from alpha rhythm? What is the prognosis suggested by this pattern as the result of hypoxia?

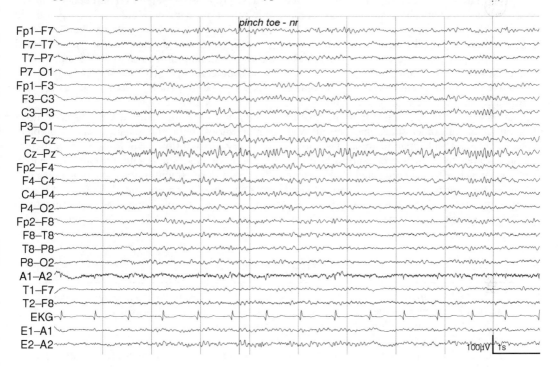

Answers: Alpha activities here are not posteriorly dominant, lack a spindle-form morphology, and are unreactive. This pattern, alpha coma, indicates poor prognosis for recovery following cerebral hypoxia.

Discussion: *Alpha coma* denotes patterns seen in profound coma that, contrary to the usual slowing of encephalopathy, consist of faster frequency activities.

Frequency of alpha coma ranges between 8 and 13 cps. Some patients demonstrate slower frequencies in the 6–7 cps range and are designated as having *theta coma*. Occasionally, low-amplitude slower frequencies are intermixed, but alpha activities are clearly the most persistent.

The amplitudes of activities are low, typically 10–25 µV and rarely >50 µV. Alpha frequencies are diffusely and symmetrically distributed and sometimes show an anterior predominance in amplitude.

The morphology and reactivity of alpha frequencies in alpha coma are characteristic: Alpha frequencies are rhythmic, monotonous, and unreactive to external stimulation or eye opening.

Alpha coma, because it shares a characteristic frequency with the normal alpha rhythm, must be differentiated from other states that present with alpha frequencies and apparent coma. The monomorphic, unreactive, diffuse or anteriorly dominant appearance of alpha coma stands in contrast to the spindle-form, posteriorly dominant, and reactive pattern of normal alpha rhythm. Two conditions present with coma-like states during which a normal alpha rhythm is recorded: (1) coma of psychiatric origin, usually catatonia and (2) "locked-in" syndrome from pontine injury, causing diffuse paralysis but sparing consciousness.

Alpha coma, although not specific for etiology, occurs most often following cerebral anoxia, such as after cardiac arrest. Rarely, alpha coma occurs as a consequence of profound sedation with barbiturates, other sedative-hypnotic agents, or from severe metabolic disarray.

The prognosis of alpha coma depends on the etiology. Following cerebral anoxia, alpha coma may be one of several patterns seen in serial recordings. Although there are rare documented cases of meaningful recovery (~4%), alpha coma following cerebral anoxia portends a grim prognosis of either impending death (~80%) or severe neurologic deficits (~16%).

Outlook from metabolic-toxic causes of alpha coma varies with the exact insult. Complete recovery may follow overdoses with sedative-hypnotic agents. Some authors point out that in drug overdose, tracings may contain enhanced beta activities or predominantly consist of higher alpha range activities than those resulting from hypoxia.

Clinical Pearls

1. Alpha coma is an EEG pattern of monomorphic, diffusely distributed, unreactive alpha-frequency activities accompanying coma and severe encephalopathy.

2. Alpha coma following cerebral anoxia marks poor prognosis for survival or meaningful neurologic recovery.

3. Alpha coma from toxic-metabolic causes correlates with severe encephalopathy but does not reliably predict poor prognosis.

4. Locked-in syndromes and catatonia may present with apparent coma and a normal alpha rhythm that must be distinguished from abnormal alpha activities in alpha coma.

REFERENCES

1. Chatrian GE: Coma, other states of unresponsiveness, and brain death. In Daly DD, Pedley TA (eds): Current Practice of Clinical Electroencephalography. New York, Raven, 1990, pp 425–487.
2. Kaplan PW, Genoud D, Ho TW, Jallon P: Etiology, neurologic correlations, and prognosis in alpha coma. Clin Neurophysiol 1999; 110:205–213.
3. Plum F, Posner JB: Pathologic physiology of signs and symptoms of coma. In Plum F, Posner JB (eds): The Diagnosis of Stupor and Coma, 3rd ed.. Philadelphia, F.A. Davis, 1982, pp 1–86.
4. Westmoreland BF, Klass DW, Sharbrough FW, Reagan TJ: Alpha-coma. Electroencephalographic, clinical, pathologic, and etiologic correlations. Arch Neurol 1975; 32:713–718.

PATIENT 89

A 23-year-old man with fulminant encephalitis and absent brainstem reflexes

A 23-year-old man presents in a coma following fulminant viral encephalitis. He is on no CNS-active medications.

Sample (a) was recorded with the patient comatose with ambiguously present corneal reflexes and decerebrate posturing. Sample (b) was recorded 24 hours later, when the patient had no brainstem reflexes. Cardiac instability prevented an apnea test. Both studies are formatted using the montage and sensitivity appropriate for an EEG cerebral death examination.

Question: Does the study during sample (b) support a diagnosis of brain death?

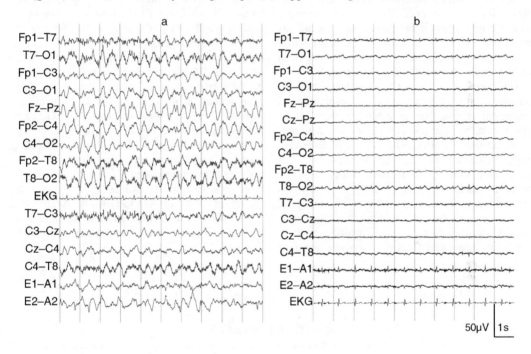

Answer: Sample *a* shows semirhythmic, approximately 25 μV delta activities. Sample *b* shows ECS. Rhythmic artifact is attributable to EKG signal. Tracing *b* is consistent with a diagnosis of brain death.

Discussion: Brain death is largely a clinical diagnosis, defined as an irreversible cessation of functions of the brain and brainstem. Confirmatory tests aid in diagnosis when neurologic exam, augmented by the apnea test, is difficult or ambiguous. Confirmatory tests include radionuclear perfusion scans, cerebral arteriography, somatosensory evoked potentials, and EEG.

ECS is the absence of discernible brain activity when recorded under strict conditions. Because the objective of the EEG *cerebral death exam* (CDE) is to demonstrate absence of activity, rather than its presence, protocols increase the possibility for cerebral activity to be faithfully recorded and to minimize erroneous conclusions regarding absence of activities. Criteria are widely accepted for adults; consensus for CDE in children falls short of wide acceptance.

Electrode placement. The montage for CDE consists of at least 8 channels, with each channel composed of nonadjacent electrode pairs, skipping frontal and parietal coronal locations so that interelectrode distance >10 cm (40% interelectrode distances in the 10–20 system). An increased interelectrode distance amplifies possible brain signal.

Calibration. To confirm the integrity of signal from patient to pen, the technologist taps each electrode in turn to record the resulting artifact. Electrode impedances must be within standard limits.

Sensitivity and duration. Recording at 2 μV/mm (or its digital peak-to-peak equivalent) for at least 30 minutes is required. The high sensitivity represents the threshold below which cerebral activity at the scalp is indistinguishable from noise.

Reactivity. Response testing to painful stimuli is mandatory.

Artifact and filters. Artifact must be identified and eliminated by the technologist, and whatever artifact remains must be identified. The ICU is rich with electrical noise, but it can usually be eliminated to a satisfactory degree. More problematic is persistent EKG artifact. Although the QRS wave is easily identifiable, the T wave can appear as rhythmic slow-wave activity. Rhythmic pulsatile artifact from underlying scalp blood flow and IV pumps may be present. Vexing, periodic artifacts, such as filling of airflow beds, deep venous thrombosis stockings, and ventilator vibration, can all appear as possible EEG bursts. Filters cannot be adjusted beyond 1 and 30 Hz.

Reversible causes of ECS include severe drug overdose and hypothermia; therefore, EEG cannot augment clinical exam in those conditions. Reversible ECS may occur during shock or other causes of cerebral hypoperfusion. Aside from these potential confounders, electrocerebral silence confirms a clinical diagnosis of brain death.

Clinical Pearls

1. ECS, when recording with accepted cerebral death examination protocols, denotes absence of cerebral activity and supports a diagnosis of brain death.
2. CDE protocol includes increased interelectrode distances, sensitivities of 2 μV/mm for at least 30 minutes, and identification and elimination of artifact.

REFERENCE
1. American Clinical Neurophysiology Society: Guideline 3: Minimum technical standards for EEG recording in suspected cerebral death. J Clin Neurophysiol 2006; 23:97–104.

PATIENT 90

A 61-year-old woman with metastatic melanoma and obtundation

A 61-year-old woman with metastatic melanoma presents with acute worsening of level of consciousness that has progressed over the previous 48 hours. On examination she is minimally responsive to tactile stimulation. A head CT with contrast shows meningeal enhancement of the tentorium and lack of hydrocephalus. She is on no medications.

The EEG is performed to rule out possible seizure activity.

Question: What are the repetitive discharges apparent in the posterior head region?

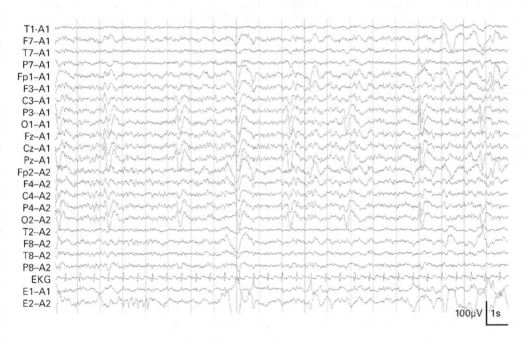

Answer: Quasi-periodic, triphasic, and polyphasic complex discharges are present, some of which appear epileptiform, with a period of recurrence at about every 3–4 seconds. They are biooccipital *periodic epileptiform discharges* (PEDs).

Discussion: Periodic discharges consist of waveforms that stand out from and interrupt background activity in a recurrent, regular pattern. Cortical activities are hardly ever truly periodic; artifact from biologic sources, such as EKG and from exogenous sources as ventilators, are more likely sources. Instead, *quasi-periodic* denotes the more typical pattern of cortical origin with a range of timings that separate discharges. For brevity, most refer to periodic discharges despite the important distinction. *PEDs* are sharp transients that recur in a periodic fashion.

Frequency and timing. The distinction between PEDS and the bursts of suppression-burst patterns is important. Bursts in suppression-bursts, like PEDs, can certainly occur periodically. Bursts, however, occur on the relative absence of background activities; PEDs usually interrupt background activities. PEDs, although often complex in morphology, imply discharges that last at the longest 1–1.5 seconds, whereas the briefest bursts in suppression-burst usually exceed 1–2 seconds in duration.

Although the timing between PEDs is variable, within an individual study the range of timings is fairly constrained. Typical PEDs recur every 1–2 seconds, with extremes between 0.5 and 5 seconds.

Although epileptiform discharges may recur periodically, a brief train of periodic discharges is not sufficient for the designation PEDs. The term should be reserved for situations in which the discharges are continuous and invariably present throughout a tracing; a 10-minute minimum has been applied in some studies.

Location. PEDS can be generalized, dominant in one region (*periodic lateralized epileptiform discharges* [PLEDs]), or occur independently or dependently in homotopic distributions (*bilateral periodic discharges* [BiPEDs]). These distinctions aid in description, but localized pathologies are not necessarily constrained to the production of PLEDS. Localized and multifocal lesions may both produce PEDs or PLEDs.

Morphology. The morphology of PEDs varies widely, ranging from sharply contoured slow wave discharges to spikes to complex, polyphasic sharp bursts. Despite the wide range of morphol-

ogies among studies, PEDs within the same study are similar (but not identical) and repetitive.

The emergence, morphology, and interdischarge interval of PEDs varies with the course and duration of the underlying cause. PEDs can emerge transiently. They appear most reliably within a day or so of the acute injury and are at their highest amplitude and complexity early. The duration of each discharge tends to be at its shortest early on. With time, the interdischarge interval increases and complexity decreases. Eventually, PEDs are usually replaced by arrhythmic delta activity, the familiar sign of chronic structural injury.

Reactivity. PEDs tend to resist attenuation with external stimuli or with endogenous state. PEDs usually occur in addition to other EEG signs of encephalopathy, so reactivity of background activities varies with the depth of loss of consciousness.

PEDs usually indicate an acute or subacute structural lesion of grey or white matter, typically both. Acute stroke is the most common cause of PEDs. CNS infections are another common cause, with herpes simplex encephalitis and Creutzfeldt-Jakob disease being other traditionally mentioned specific causes. Occasionally, metabolic disorders will provoke PEDs in those with existing localized pathology.

Seizures commonly coexist with PEDs. Even though seizures and PEDs seemingly go hand-in-hand, PEDs are not necessarily predictive of future epileptic seizures. Seizures and PEDs probably represent the coexisting signs of acute brain injury, rather than evidence of the future risk of seizures. In other words, PEDs are an epileptiform pattern that is not clearly epileptogenic. An important refinement to that last statement is that PEDs may indicate ongoing seizure activity. PEDs occur in end-stage status epilepticus, in experimental animal models of epilepsy, and may represent the ictal discharge in patients with nonconvulsive status epilepticus.

In this patient's case, the EEG finding of biooccipital PEDs leads physicians to acquire an MRI that demonstrates bilateral posterior invasion of metastatic lesions. Malignant and rapid invasion of tumor is another etiology associated with PEDs.

Clinical Pearls

    1. PEDs are continuously present, poorly reactive, periodic epileptiform discharges.

    2. PEDs usually denote acute destructive lesions.

    3. Although seizures may occur during the acute brain lesion that causes PEDs, PEDs are not predictive of future risk of epileptic seizures.

    4. PEDs are one of the forms of chronic or ongoing ictal discharges and can be seen in nonconvulsive status epilepticus.

REFERENCES

1. Chong DJ, Hirschl J: Which EEG patterns warrant treatment in the clinically ill? Reviewing the evidence for treatment of periodic epileptiform discharges and related patterns. J Clin Neurophysiol 2005; 22:79–91.
2. Garcia-Morales I, Garcia MT, Galan-Davila L, et al: Periodic lateralized epileptiform discharges: Etiology, clinical aspects, seizures, and evolution in 130 patients. J Clin Neurophysiol 2002; 19(2):172–177.
3. Pohlmann-Eden B, Hoch DB, Cochius JI, Chiappa KH: Periodic lateralized epileptiform discharges—A critical review. J Clin Neurophysiol 1996; 13(6):519–530.

PATIENT 91

A 70-year-old man with fever, confusion, and aphasia

An EEG is requested for a 70-year-old man with several days of fever followed by confusion and expressive aphasia. Medications include broad-spectrum antibiotics and acyclovir.

The recording is made with the patient awake.

Questions: What are the EEG findings? What is the most likely diagnosis given the clinical information and EEG findings?

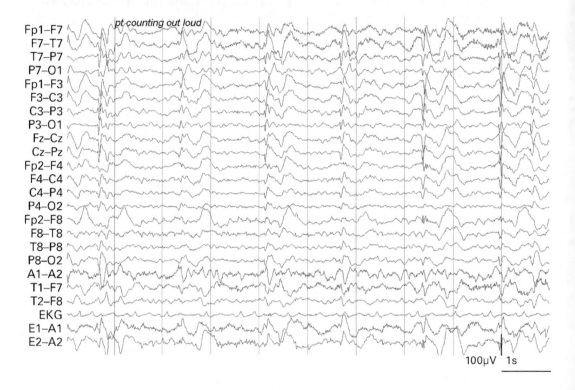

Periodic Epileptiform Discharges

Answers: Background activities consist of arrhythmic delta and theta activities. PLEDs are present with greater involvement of the left hemisphere with phase-reversal variably present in the posterior temporal region. The EEG supports a diagnosis of acute herpes simplex viral encephalitis.

Discussion: Historically, EEG was an important tool in the diagnosis of possible herpes simplex viral encephalitis (HSVE). PLEDs, in the setting of fever and delirium or lethargy, occurred earlier and was a more specific finding than changes on head CT in early HSVE. PLEDs, therefore, were evidence that often paved the way to a diagnostic brain biopsy.

The availability of effective therapy for HSVE, however, modified the need for acute EEG in the diagnostic and treatment plan. Currently, patients with suspected HSVE are routinely treated with the antiviral agent acyclovir while awaiting detection of HSV in the plasma or *cerebrospinal fluid* (CSF) through the use of the *polymerase chain reaction* (PCR) test.

Nevertheless, EEG does have an adjunctive and useful role in the current process.

First, the findings of PLEDs in suspected HSVE remain a sensitive test. For example, in neonates with HSVE, PLEDs or other focal abnormalities on EEG are present in over 80%, compared to other signs, such as HSV rash (40%) or MRI abnormalities (65%) within 12 days of clinical onset.

PLEDs may have a prognostic value in PCR-proven HSVE. PLEDs are associated with worse neurologic outcome. Past studies also showed that abnormal background activities in conjunction with PLEDs also correlated with poor neurologic outcome, but this later finding may not hold true in the age of acyclovir treatment.

In this patient's case, the PCR test was positive for HSV. The left temporal PLEDs were found in the third day after clinical onset of fever. A subsequent EEG repeated on hospital day 10 (13 days after onset) showed left temporal arrhythmic delta activity. Repeat EEGs are recommended to document the gradual evolution of PLEDs.

Clinical Pearls

1. PLEDs are an important adjunct in the evaluation and treatment of herpes simplex viral encephalitis.

2. PLEDs appear earlier in the time course of herpetic encephalitis than neuroimaging.

3. The persistence and presence of PLEDs in herpetic encephalitis are associated with worse outcome in acyclovir-treated patients.

REFERENCES
1. Kimberlin DW, Jacobs RF, Powell DA, et al: Natural history of neonatal herpes simplex virus infections in the acyclovir era. Pediatrics 2001; 108:223–229.
2. Siren J, Seppalainen AM, Launes J: Is EEG useful in assessing patients with acute encephalitis treated with acyclovir? Electroencephalogr Clin Neurophysiol 1998; 107(4):296–301.

PATIENT 92

A 71-year-old man with rapidly progressive memory loss and somnolence

A 71-year-old man presents with rapidly progressive memory loss, personality changes, and somnolence. He has a history of bipolar disorder and chronic obstructive pulmonary disease (COPD). He is noted to have intermittent shaking of the left arm. Medications include lithium and valproate.

The EEG is performed with the patient awake. There are no EEG correlates to left arm movements.

Questions: What is the predominant EEG finding? What group of encephalopathies does this sample suggest in the setting of rapidly progressive dementia?

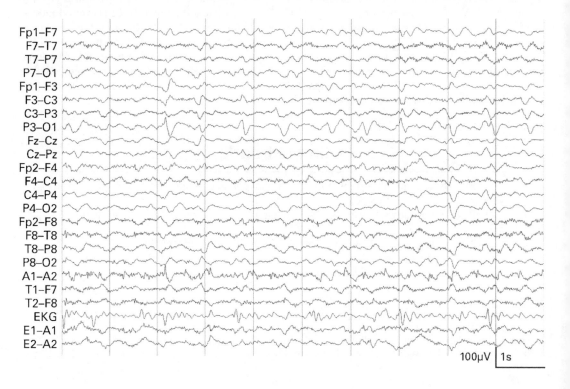

Periodic Epileptiform Discharges

Answers: PLEDs are present in the left centrotemporal region, occasionally involving the contralateral hemisphere. In the setting of rapidly progressive dementia, PLEDs suggest prion infection (Creutzfeldt-Jakob disease).

Discussion: The most common human prion disease is *Creutzfeldt-Jakob disease* (CJD), which accounts for about 85% of prion infections. The primary symptoms of CJD are a rapidly progressive dementia, myoclonus, and variable evidence of multifocal neurologic disease.

The EEG in CJD typically shows PEDs or PLEDs on abnormally slow background activity. Myoclonus coincides with PEDs, but treatment with anticonvulsants does not necessarily resolve either. The EEG has reasonable specificity and sensitivity (67% and 87%, respectively) in predicting the typical spongiform degeneration seen on autopsy or biopsy. The main shortcoming of EEG in the diagnosis of CJD is that, like the usual course of PEDs in structural injuries, PEDs occur transiently and may be absent in early stages of the disease.

PEDs occur about 2 months after the first clinical changes, usually coinciding with the development of myoclonus and akinetic mutism. One study found that FIRDA often preceded onset of PEDs and myoclonus and should guide recommendations for repeat study. Repeat recordings can greatly improve the chances of a positive diagnosis, so that 90% of patients with CJD at one point of their illness demonstrate PEDs.

Other prion diseases lack a clear association with PEDs, so that lack of PEDs does not provide evidence against such variants as fatal familial insomnia or the human form of bovine spongiform encephalopathy.

One concern is the iatrogenic spread of prion disease with the reuse of EEG electrodes. Because the prion protein is resistant to common, vigorous methods of sterilization, EEG electrodes are not reused if the clinical question is possible CJD. An exception to this rule is that electrodes may be autoclaved and bleached for later reuse for an individual patient.

Other infectious agents besides CJD can cause PEDs. *Subacute sclerosing panencephalitis* (SSPE) is a chronic measles encephalitis of childhood that is now rare in the United States because of immunization. As in CJD, PEDs appear in the setting of dementia and myoclonus. Sometimes the interval between periodic complexes can be quite prolonged in SSPE.

Clinical Pearls

1. Findings of PEDs in the setting of dementia and myoclonus are suggestive of prion disease.
2. Electrodes are not reused if the differential diagnosis is prion disease.
3. In children, SSPE should join the differential diagnosis, especially if the inter-complex interval is prolonged.

REFERENCES

1. Aguglia U, Farnarier G, Tinuper P, et al: Subacute spongiform encephalopathy with periodic paroxysmal activities: Clinical evolution and serial EEG findings in 20 cases. Clin Electroencephalogr 1987; 18(3):147–158.
2. Chiofalo N, Fuentes A, Galvez S: Serial EEG findings in 27 cases of Creutzfeldt-Jakob disease. Arch Neurol 1980; 37(3):143–145.
3. Hansen HC, Zschocke S, Sturenburg HJ, Kunze K: Clinical changes and EEG patterns preceding the onset of periodic sharp wave complexes in Creutzfeldt-Jakob disease. Acta Neurol Scand 1998; 97(2):99–106.

PATIENT 93

An 83-year-old woman with recurrent confusion and seizures

An emergent EEG is requested to evaluate delirium in an 83-year-old, right-handed woman with a history of an old left cerebral hemorrhage. She presents with a seizure involving the right arm and the face. She was seen a week before in the emergency department with confusion that spontaneously improved with no evidence of metabolic abnormalities or new stroke. Symptoms recurred intermittently since. On this admission, she cannot follow commands on exam.

The EEG is obtained in the emergency department with the patient awake. Medications are unknown.

Questions: What are the two locations of periodic discharges in this sample? Does this recording refute the diagnosis of delirium?

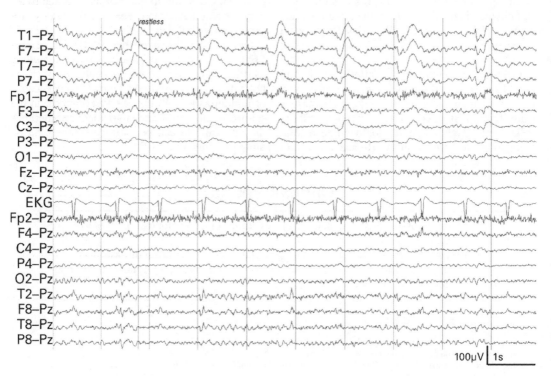

Periodic Epileptiform Discharges

Answers: PLEDs with a frequency of 1.5–2 cps occur broadly across the left anterior temporal region. Periodic activity across the right temporal region arises from EKG artifact. The relatively fast activities apparent in background activity argue against a metabolic encephalopathy. "Delirium" in this case may be referable to a receptive aphasia rather than a bihemispheric encephalopathy.

Discussion: This patient's case illustrates the use of EEG in aiding the diagnosis of neurologic syndromes that can present with similar presentations. In this case, waxing and waning attention and inability to follow commands could result from either a diffuse encephalopathy causing delirium or focal dysfunction of the dominant hemisphere inducing a receptive aphasia.

This tracing shows prominent left temporal PLEDs and independent right temporal periodic discharges. The EKG channel, however, demonstrates that the latter are EKG artifact rather than independent PLEDs. Another hint for proper distinction between the two is that left temporal PLEDs occur in a quasi-periodic pattern every 1.5–2 seconds, but right temporal artifact is truly periodic at the cardiac sinus rhythm.

The background activities consist of poorly organized theta activities across the left hemisphere and 9–10 cps, posteriorly dominant alpha activities across the right hemisphere (with occasional low-amplitude, posteriorly dominant alpha activities apparent on the left as well). Although alpha rhythm is not explicitly demonstrated with eye opening or closure, in this sample, the frequencies and distribution can be considered presumptive alpha rhythm.

Left temporal PLEDs and mild slowing of background activities of wakefulness across the left hemisphere suggest acute localized dysfunction. The findings here are not specific enough to determine whether her symptoms are referable to an acute destructive lesion, such as new stroke, an ongoing complex partial seizure (complex partial status epilepticus), or a combination of the two.

This patient's syndrome spontaneously resolved several hours after the EEG. A head CT showed no evidence of new infarct or hemorrhage. With the differential diagnosis, including transient ischemic attacks and recurrent complex partial seizures/nonconvulsive status epilepticus, she was treated with antiplatelet therapies and anticonvulsant medications (carbamazepine).

Clinical Pearls

1. Accurate interpretation of periodic discharges requires the use of an EKG channel.
2. PLEDs can represent an acute structural lesion or ongoing seizure activity.

REFERENCE

1. Chong DJ, Hirschl J: Which EEG patterns warrant treatment in the clinically ill? Reviewing the evidence for treatment of periodic epileptiform discharges and related patterns. J Clin Neurophysiol 2005; 22:79–91.
2. Kaplan PW: Nonconvulsive status epilepticus in the emergency room. Epilepsia 1996; 37(7):643–650.

PATIENT 94

A 52-year-old man with epilepsy found inattentive and disoriented

An EEG is requested to evaluate possible ongoing seizure activity in a 52-year-old man with a history of idiopathic generalized seizures who was found confused. The patient is taking phenytoin and valproate.

Two 20-second samples are shown. During the first, baseline sample ("before diazepam"), the patient is awake, inattentive, and disoriented; during the second ("after diazepam"), the patient is more alert and attentive but remains disoriented.

Questions: Describe the baseline EEG. Do the responses to the ongoing treatment confirm a diagnosis of nonconvulsive status epilepticus?

before diazepam

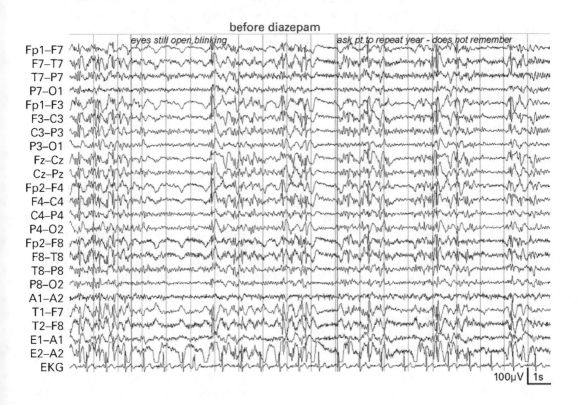

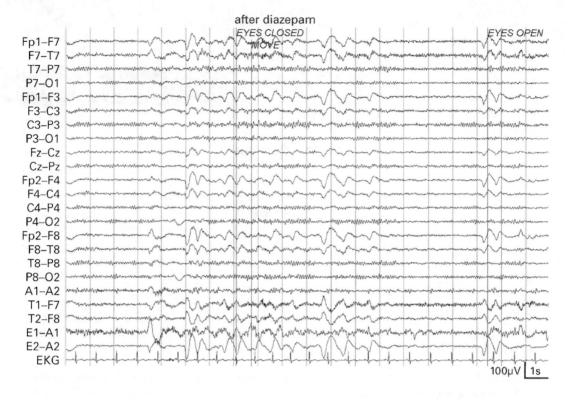

after diazepam

EYES CLOSED
MOVE

EYES OPEN

100μV | 1s

Answers: The baseline EEG depicts recurrent bursts of rhythmic multiple spike discharges on background activities of diffusely distributed alpha activity. Bursts of multiple spike activity resolve coinciding with clinical improvement. Resolution of clinical impairment and electrographic seizure activity following anticonvulsant treatment is diagnostic of *nonconvulsive status epilepticus* (NCSE).

Discussion: NCSE is a state of continuous electrographic seizures lasting longer than 30 minutes that is not accompanied by clinically obvious motor activity. Instead, a wide range of impairments of consciousness accompanies electrical status epilepticus, from a vague, subjective discomfort, to impaired attention, lethargy, waxing and waning delirium or clouded consciousness, stupor, or coma. Sometimes simple, repetitive, and subtle motor activities are present, such as beating lateral nystagmus-like activity, facial or periorbital clonus, repetitive posturing, or changes in tone.

Henri Gastaut is attributed with the observation that there are as many different types of status epilepticus as there are types of seizures. Generalized *convulsive status epilepticus* (CSE), although the most common of status epilepticus syndromes, is mainly a clinical diagnosis; EEG is not required, and, in field conditions, is often not emergently available. However, 14–20% of patients with CSE continue to have EEG evidence of ictal activity (i.e., NCSE) despite resolution of clinical signs of seizures. The role of

EEG in CSE, therefore, is to confirm the resolution of ongoing seizure activity in those patients who fail to improve following cessation of clinical convulsions and to monitor the success of ongoing therapy.

In this case, the patient had known idiopathic generalized epilepsy, emphasizing that NCSE can be divided in two basic categories:

Absence status epilepticus (i.e., ictal stupor, spike-wave stupor) consists of prolonged episodes of absence seizures that are accompanied by continuous generalized discharges. It is usually seen in patients with idiopathic generalized epilepsies. Beyond the morbidity of impaired consciousness, outcome is thought to be relatively benign.

Partial status epilepticus (i.e., subtle status epilepticus, complex partial status epilepticus) consists of prolonged focal or regional ictal discharges of various morphologies. Secondary generalization may occur. In contrast to absence status epilepticus, acute brain injury may cause seizures, and outcome is often tied to the underlying etiology. In addition, complex partial status epilepticus in experimental animal models causes permanent neuronal injury. In humans, complex partial status epilepticus is associated with subsequent cognitive impairment.

Although EEG is required to make the diagnosis of NCSE, the ongoing ictal discharge often does not cleanly fall into localized or generalized seizure patterns, and one may evolve into the other during prolonged episodes. Adding to the challenge is that ictal discharges are often difficult to distinguish from other rhythmic, nonictal activity, such as PEDs or triphasic waves.

Patients who meet the following criteria have definite NCSE:

1. Clinical state is impaired from baseline and is present continuously or intermittently without full recovery for 30 minutes or more.
2. EEG shows ongoing electrographic seizure activity.
3. Interictal or postictal EEG shows IEDs.
4. Both impaired clinical state and electrographic seizure activity improve or resolve following treatment with anticonvulsant medications.

Of these criteria, the last is often the most difficult to fulfill. First, clinical improvement may be subtle, so that preictal and postictal testing should strive to document consistent observations in attention, level of consciousness, and activities.

Second, postictal state can be prolonged following status epilepticus. Outside of those patients with absence status epilepticus after which recovery can be instantaneous, clinical improvement lags behind electrographic resolution. Third, the underlying etiology of status epilepticus may independently cause impairment from seizure activity, so that the states of comatose patients rarely change in the course of a routine EEG. Serial or continuous prolonged EEGs, supplemented with clinical examination, may, with time, demonstrate clinical improvement.

Drug administration in the diagnosis of NCSE is often out of the hands of the interpreting electroencephalographer, but the team of physicians should be aware that medication and administration may aid in a clear diagnosis. The agents most useful for acute administration during EEG in the diagnosis of NCSE are the benzodiazepines. Lorazepam is the favored agent because of efficacy demonstrated in the multicenter study of treatment of CSE. Other electroencephalographers prefer diazepam or midazolam for *diagnosis*, rather than *treatment* because of more rapid dispersion into the CNS. Whichever the specific benzodiazepine, it should be administered intravenously and flushed rapidly to induce a quick and unambiguous change in the ongoing EEG. Consistent clinical testing establishes the patient's best performance before and after empiric treatment.

Clinical Pearls

1. NCSE consists of continuous electrographic seizure activity with the clinical accompaniment of impairment or loss of consciousness.

2. Partial and generalized NCSE are the two main subtypes, but they can be poorly distinguished on EEG.

3. Diagnosis of NCSE relies upon clinical testing, empiric benzodiazepine treatment, and clear documentation of the patient's best response or state before and after treatment.

REFERENCES

1. Craven W, Faught E, Kuzniecky R, et al: Residual electrographic status epilepticus after control of overt electrical seizures [abstract]. Epilepsia 1995; 36:S46.
2. Fountain NB, Lothman EW: Pathophysiology of status epilepticus. J Clin Neurophysiol 1995; 12(4):326–342.
3. Granner MA, Lee SI: Nonconvulsive status epilepticus: EEG analysis in a large series. Epilepsia 1994; 35(1):42–47.
4. Kaplan PW: Nonconvulsive status epilepticus in the emergency room. Epilepsia 1996; 37(7):643–650.
5. Kirby D, Fountain NB, Quigg M: Standardized mental status testing for nonconvulsive status epilepticus. Am J Electroneurodiagnostic Technol 2004; 44(3):199–201.
6. Krumholz A, Sung GY, Fisher RS, et al: Complex partial status epilepticus accompanied by serious morbidity mortality. Neurology 1995; 45(8):1499–1504.
7. Quigg M, Shneker B, Domer P: Current practice in administration and clinical criteria of emergent EEG. J Clin Neurophysiol 2001; 18(2):162–165.
8. Scholtes FB, Renier WG, Meinardi H: Non-convulsive status epilepticus: Causes, treatment, outcome in 65 patients. J Neurosurg Neurol Psychiatry 1994; 61:93–95.

9. Treiman DM, Meyers PD, Walton NY, et al: A comparison of four treatments for generalized convulsive status epilepticus. Veterans Affairs Status Epilepticus Cooperative Study Group. N Engl J Med 1998; 339:792–798.
10. Young GB, Jordan KG, Doig GS: An assessment of nonconvulsive seizures in the intensive care unit using continuous EEG monitoring: An investigation of variables associated with mortality. Neurology 1996; 47(1):83–89.

PATIENT 95

A 60-year-old woman with decline in mental status

An EEG is requested to determine the etiology of decline in the level of consciousness in a 60-year-old woman with a history of lung transplant. She has no laboratory evidence of toxic-metabolic encephalopathy. No convulsive seizures are witnessed, but persistent leftward eye deviation and myoclonus are present. She is taking immunosuppressive and antihypertensive medications.

The study demonstrates nearly continuous runs of 2–3 cps triphasic waves of varying morphology that are often generalized but sometimes have higher amplitudes in the vertex and left parasagittal regions. External stimulation does not change the patterns, and there is no detectable anterior-posterior lag among triphasic waves. Two samples are shown, one before administration of 5 mg IV diazepam ("before diazepam") and another about 1 minute after administration ("after diazepam"). All clinical movements cease during the second sample.

Question: What is the diagnosis?

before diazepam

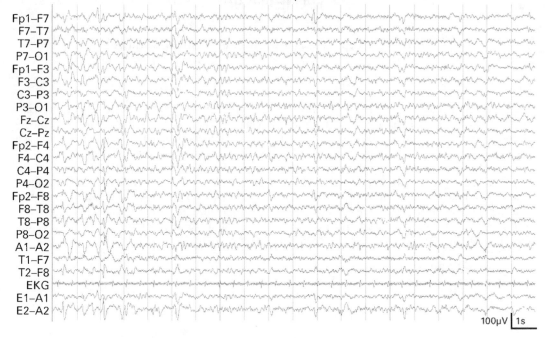

Fp1–F7
F7–T7
T7–P7
P7–O1
Fp1–F3
F3–C3
C3–P3
P3–O1
Fz–Cz
Cz–Pz
Fp2–F4
F4–C4
C4–P4
P4–O2
Fp2–F8
F8–T8
T8–P8
P8–O2
A1–A2
T1–F7
T2–F8
EKG
E1–A1
E2–A2

100µV | 1s

Answer: Clinical and electrographic NCSE marked by clinical improvement coinciding with resolution of 2.75–3 cps diffusely distributed sharp-wave/slow-wave complexes with a triphasic morphology.

Discussion: The ictal discharges present in NCSE can be easy to confuse with other rhythmic activities that do not represent seizure activity. Triphasic waves of toxic-metabolic or ictal origins may be indistinguishable from each other.

The diagnostic criteria for ictal discharges in NCSE are controversial, but some guidelines exist. Proposed primary and secondary criteria are as follows:

Primary Criteria

1. Repetitive generalized or focal spikes, sharp waves, spike-and-wave, or sharp-and-slow wave complexes at more than 3 per second.
2. Repetitive generalized or focal spikes, sharp waves, spike-and-wave, or sharp-and-slow wave complexes at fewer than 3 per second and secondary criterion no. 4.
3. Sequential rhythmic waves and secondary criteria 1, 2, and 3 with or without secondary criterion no. 4.

Secondary Criteria

1. Incrementing onset: increase in voltage or increase or slowing of frequency.
2. Decrementing offset: decrease in voltage or frequency.
3. Post-discharge slowing or voltage attenuation.
4. Significant improvement in clinical state or baseline EEG after intravenous *antiepileptic drug* (AED).

Of course, the range of potential ictal discharges allowed by such flexible criteria is vast. In this patient's case, rhythmic sharp and slow-wave complexes (with a triphasic morphology) with a frequency just under 3 cps (primary criterion no. 2) attenuated with benzodiazepines (secondary criterion no. 4). This tracing also demonstrated rhythmic evolution of triphasic waves as the EEG progressed, fulfilling secondary criteria no.1 and no. 2, but this finding is not discernible in these brief samples.

Note that attenuation of rhythmic activity with benzodiazepines is not proof of NCSE, just supportive of the diagnosis. Patients with triphasic waves of metabolic-toxic origin can also show resolution of triphasic waves with benzodiazepines, supposedly on the basis of transiently worsened encephalopathy from sedation.

Clinical examination, therefore, remains an important component in the use of benzodiazepines in the diagnosis of NCSE. Only with clinical improvement in correlation with electrographic resolution is there a definitive diagnosis of NCSE.

Clinical Pearl

Rhythmic discharges of ictal origin must be distinguished from those of nonictal origin on the basis of morphology, evolution, reactivity, and clinical and electrographical responses to anticonvulsant medications.

REFERENCES

1. Chong DJ, Hirschl J: Which EEG patterns warrant treatment in the clinically ill? Reviewing the evidence for treatment of periodic epileptiform discharges and related patterns. J Clin Neurophysiol 2005; 22:79–91.
2. Fountain NB, Waldman WA: Effects of benzodiazepines on triphasic waves: Implications for nonconvulsive status epilepticus. J Clin Neurophysiol 2001; 18(4):345–352.
3. Young GB, Jordan KG, Doig GS: An assessment of nonconvulsive seizures in the intensive care unit using continuous EEG monitoring: An investigation of variables associated with mortality. Neurology 1996; 47(1):83–89.

PATIENT 96

A 74-year-old man in a coma after cardiac arrest

An EEG is requested to evaluate possible NCSE in a patient who has two convulsive seizures and does not clinically improve in level of consciousness 4 hours after the last event. Seizures occur after cardiac arrest, resuscitation, and acute myocardial infarction. His medications include phenytoin and lorazepam.

The baseline EEG is recorded at bedside with patient comatose and ventilated ("before diazepam"). "Arms extended" in the second sample ("after diazepam") corresponds to decerebrate posturing evoked by painful stimulation, a response not present during the baseline recording.

Questions: What are the baseline findings? Does the second sample confirm a diagnosis of NCSE?

before diazepam

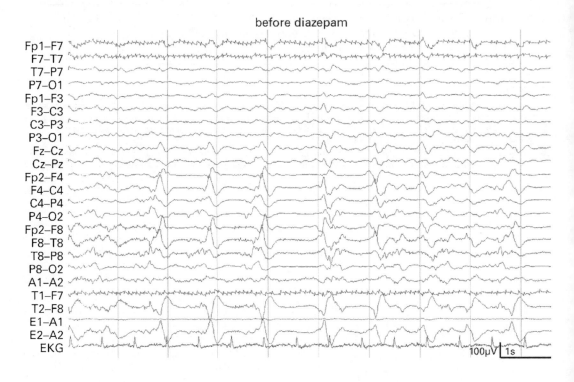

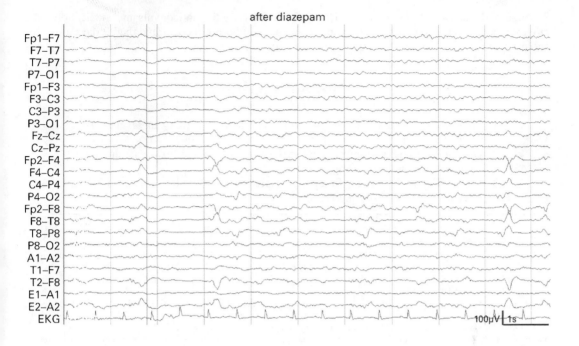

after diazepam

Fp1–F7
F7–T7
T7–P7
P7–O1
Fp1–F3
F3–C3
C3–P3
P3–O1
Fz–Cz
Cz–Pz
Fp2–F4
F4–C4
C4–P4
P4–O2
Fp2–F8
F8–T8
T8–P8
P8–O2
A1–A2
T1–F7
T2–F8
E1–A1
E2–A2
EKG

100µV 1s

Answers: PLEDs with a periodicity of approximately 1 per second appear across the right hemisphere on suppressed background activities. Clinical improvement and electrographic resolution following administration of benzodiazepines confirm a diagnosis of NCSE.

Discussion: In the paradigm provided by animal models of status epilepticus, PEDs represent the late effect of chronic, untreated CSE. As CSE progresses, discrete clinical seizures merge to form waxing and waning obtundation. Bursts of ictal activity, originally separated by abnormal background activity, progress to nearly continuous rhythmic ictal discharges. If allowed to continue, clinical seizure activity may evolve to stupor or coma without clear convulsions. The electrographic end stage in this process is PEDs.

On the other hand, PEDS occur late in experimental status epilepticus. PEDS may represent electrographic evidence of acute neuronal injury following prolonged seizures. Thus, PEDs may represent the injury resulting from long-lasting seizures. Subsequent findings in humans with severe status epilepticus, however, document that PEDs resolve with successful anticonvulsant therapy, providing evidence that PEDs are ictal.

Clinical and experimental work have converged to suggest that PEDs in a comatose patient should lead to the diagnosis of status epilepticus, even if clinical movements are absent or are extremely subtle. In this light, NCSE is a potentially treatable cause of coma that requires an

emergent EEG to make the diagnosis. The main problem facing clinicians is that no clear markers in the EEG itself, divorced from clinical information, reliably separate PEDs of ictal origin from those that designate acute, destructive lesions. PEDs of ictal origin may show evidence of spatial and temporal evolution: Amplitude or frequency may wax and wane, or spontaneously stop only to recur, and PEDs may show variable location. PEDs of ictal origin should attenuate with a trial of anticonvulsant medication. PEDs from acute structural lesions, on the other hand, remain continuous, poorly reactive, localized to one distribution, and do not attenuate with anticonvulsant medication.

In this patient's case, witnessed convulsions evolved to a continuous state of coma and NCSE. Up to 20% of convulsive status epilepticus continues to have NCSE following resolution of clinical movements. Residual NCSE following convulsive status epilepticus is a poor prognostic sign, with 65% dying within 30 days of presentation. In comparison, only 27% of patients died whose CSE resolved without evidence of NCSE. An EEG is recommended to determine the electrographic success of treatment of status epilepticus if the patient shows no evidence of clinical recovery following treatment. Despite the successful treatment of electrographic seizure activity with anticonvulsant medication, the patient did not recover and died 2 days after this recording.

Clinical Pearls

1. PEDs may represent ongoing electrographic seizure activity in severe seizures and encephalopathies.

2. Distinguishing ictal from nonictal PEDs requires clinical examination and adjunctive anticonvulsant use during the EEG.

3. An EEG should be done following resolution of CSE, if there is no clinical improvement to rule out ongoing NCSE.

REFERENCES

1. Chong DJ, Hirschl J: Which EEG patterns warrant treatment in the clinically ill? Reviewing the evidence for treatment of periodic epileptiform discharges and related patterns. J Clin Neurophysiol 2005; 22:79–91.
2. Craven W, Faught E, Kuzniecky R, et al: Residual electrographic status epilepticus after control of overt electrical seizures [abstract]. Epilepsia 1995; 36:S46.
3. Quigg M, Schneker B, Domer P: Current practice administration of emergent EEG. J Clin Neurophysiol 2001; 18:162–165.
4. Treiman DM, Meyers PD, Walton NY, et al: A comparison of four treatments for generalized convulsive status epilepticus. Veterans Affairs Status Epilepticus Cooperative Study Group. N Engl J Med 1998; 339:792–798.
5. Treiman DM, Walton NY, Kendrick C: A progressive sequence of electroencephalographic changes during generalized convulsive status epilepticus. Epilepsy Res 1990; 5(1):49–60.

PATIENT 97

A 71-year-old man with stupor and asterixis

A 71-year-old man with hepatitis presents with worsening confusion and negative myoclonus (asterixis). An EEG is requested to evaluate possible NCSE. He takes no CNS-active medication.

The recording is performed with the patient lethargic and intermittently trembling. The first sample ("before diazepam") shows 20 seconds during which external stimulation is performed. The second 10-second sample ("during injection") shows the patient during unstimulated rest during administration of intravenous diazepam. The third sample ("after diazepam") shows activities 20 minutes after the diazepam is flushed. The patient shows no clinical changes throughout the study.

Questions: What are the patterns in the first and second samples? What are the activities in the third sample? Are the findings compatible with NCSE?

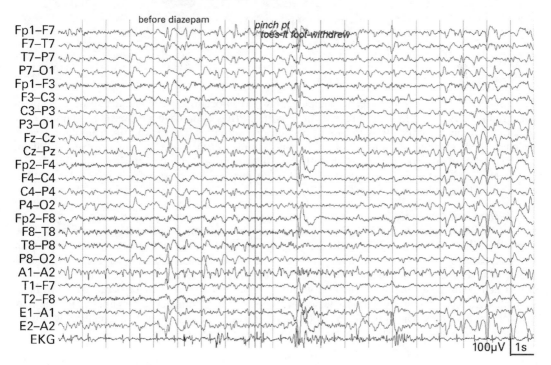

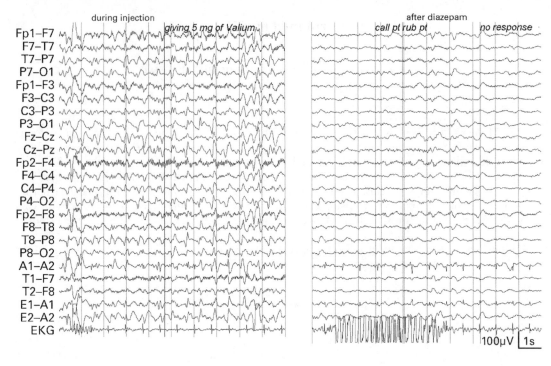

during injection   giving 5 mg of Valium   after diazepam   call pt rub pt   no response

100µV   1s

Answers: The first and second samples show PEDs occurring at a frequency of 1–2 cps on background activities of low-amplitude theta activities. PEDs often have a triphasic morphology and sometimes occur rhythmically with loss of background activities. During the first sample, activities attenuate with external stimulation. In the third sample, PEDs have largely resolved following administration of diazepam. Despite the effect of diazepam on periodic activities, the finding that they resolve with stimulation suggests that PEDs/triphasic waves arise from metabolic or toxic encephalopathies rather than ongoing NCSE.

Discussion: One procedure to help the diagnosis of NCSE is administration of anticonvulsants during the EEG. Resolution of rhythmic EEG activity supports, but does not prove, a diagnosis of NCSE. The reason for this cautious interpretation is that benzodiazepines attenuate triphasic waves of toxic-metabolic origin by further decreasing level of consciousness. The only time benzodiazepine administration is diagnostic in NCSE is when clinical improvement accompanies resolution of the rhythmic discharge on EEG.

In this patient's case, external stimulation attenuates triphasic waves (sample "before diazepam"), suggesting that rhythmic activity is reactive and unlikely to be ictal. The physician decided to administer diazepam, despite the findings of reactivity because attenuation was not a consistent response.

Clinical Pearls

---

1. Diagnosis of NCSE requires evaluation of all of the findings at hand, including patient responses to reactivity and to diazepam.

2. Administration of benzodiazepines may resolve triphasic waves by inducing a transient exacerbation in encephalopathy.

REFERENCE

1. Chong DJ, Hirschl J: Which EEG patterns warrant treatment in the clinically ill? Reviewing the evidence for treatment of periodic epileptiform discharges and related patterns. J Clin Neurophysiol 2005; 22:79–91.
2. Fountain NB, Waldman WA: Effects of benzodiazepines on triphasic waves: Implications for nonconvulsive status epilepticus. J Clin Neurophysiol 2001; 18(4):345–352.

PATIENT 98

An 8-year-old boy with static encephalopathy and recurrent myoclonus

An 8-year-old boy presents with spells of bilateral arm and trunk jerking and no clear alteration of consciousness. He has severe static encephalopathy after viral meningoencephalitis and is blind and quadriplegic. He takes no CNS-active medications.

The EEG is obtained with the patient awake and with continuous, repetitive jerks of the trunk.

Question: What is the origin of periodic discharges in this sample?

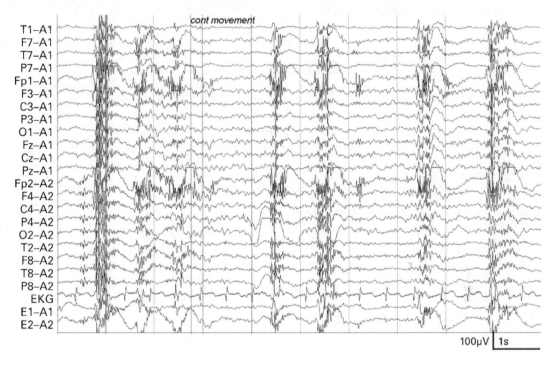

Answer: Periodic bursts of diffuse muscle activity occur upon low-amplitude, suppressed background activities.

Discussion: Myoclonus can have cortical, subcortical, or spinal localizations.

Cortical myoclonus is sometimes called *epileptic myoclonus* and is accompanied by evidence of epileptiform discharges.

Subcortical or *spinal myoclonus* (also known as *nonepileptic myoclonus*) often has no evidence of epileptic activity. Special recording techniques that record samples of EEG and are time-locked to episodes of myoclonus can confirm the sequential order of epileptic potentials to myoclonic jerks. With the use of time-locked recording and sample-averaging (a technique that increases signal strength by averaging reproducible signal over random noise), the timing of myoclonus versus cortical activity can be quantified.

Responses to anticonvulsants in myoclonus can be unpredictable because clinical symptoms can respond but electrographic discharges may not.

In this patient's case, the bursts of electrical activity consist of muscle and movement artifact. Such findings often support a diagnosis of non-epileptic myoclonus, but the present tracing is ambiguous because of the masking of possible cortical potentials by artifact.

Clinical Pearls

1. Myoclonus may be classified by routine EEG into epileptic and nonepileptic myoclonus.
2. Persistent movement or dystonia may mask EEG findings with artifact.

REFERENCE

1. Niedermeyer E, Riley T: Myoclonus the electroencephalogram: A review [112 refs]. Clin Electroencephalogr 1979; 10(2):75–95.
2. Shibasaki H, Yamashita Y, Tobimatsu S, Neshige R: Electroencephalographic correlates of myoclonus. Adv Neurol 1986; 43:357–372.

PATIENT 99

A 45-year-old man with a coma and myoclonus

A 45-year-old man presents with a coma and myoclonus. He has hepatitis C and alcoholic cirrhosis with recent pneumonia, sepsis, and upper gastrointestinal (GI) hemorrhage. Rhythmic jerking begins on the second day of coma. Listed medications include lorazepam drip.

The EEG is obtained while the patient is sedated, intubated, and comatose. Continuous generalized jerking is present at baseline (''periodic myoclonus'') and is mostly absent (except for residual facial clonus) after administration of vecuronium (''after vecuronium'').

Questions: From interpretation of the baseline sample only, what are the possible sources of the bursts? What does administration of vecuronium accomplish in the interpretation? Is there evidence of status epilepticus?

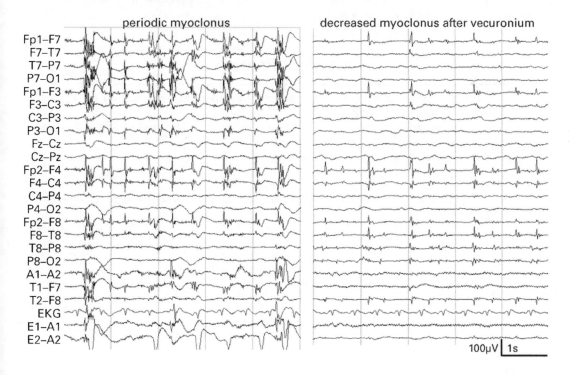

Answers: Quasi-periodic bursts of extremely sharp activities, in the first sample, can be either bursts of muscle artifact or PEDs. Vecuronium, a paralytic agent, resolves all-but-residual myoclonus. The EEG responds similarly, showing near resolution of bursts (later on, all muscular and apparent EEG activity resolves, but worsening electrical noise prevents its presentation here). Paralysis confirms that quasi-periodic bursts are artifact, leaving low-amplitude, diffusely distributed delta activity. The diagnosis is nonepileptic myoclonus.

Discussion: Vecuronium and other paralytic agents can aid interpretation of the EEG by removing the obscuring effect of muscle artifact. Of course, paralytic agents can be administered only in comatose or thoroughly sedated subjects to prevent the possibility of conscious paralysis, a potentially terrifying experience.

Paralytic agents or, more precisely, those who use paralytic agents, have earned poor reputations with those charged in diagnosis of status epilepticus. Paralytic agents are often used emergently to aid in the establishment and maintenance of the airway in violently convulsing patients. Occasionally, however, one may use paralytic agents to "treat" persisting convulsive movements, forgetting that electrical seizure activity may persist despite neuromuscular blockade. Iatrogenic paralysis induced after witnessed seizure activity is a clear indication for emergent EEG to ensure against iatrogenic NCSE.

In this patient's case, no cerebral activities coincide with myoclonus, best classifying the syndrome as nonepileptic myoclonus.

Clinical Pearls

1. Paralytic agents may allow interpretation of EEG in tracings obscured by muscle artifact in appropriate patients.

2. Iatrogenic paralysis following a witnessed seizure requires a follow-up EEG to confirm resolution of electrical seizure activity.

REFERENCE

1. Quigg M, Shneker B, Domer P: Current practice in administration and clinical criteria of emergent EEG. J Clin Neurophysiol 2001; 18(2):162–165.

PATIENT 100

A 74-year-old man with a coma and myoclonus following cardiac arrest

An EEG to aid in ongoing treatment of CSE is requested for a 74-year-old man after cardiac resuscitation for asystolic arrest. He has generalized convulsive seizures, confirmed by witnesses, immediately after resuscitation. After emergent treatment with lorazepam, he continues to have myoclonic jerks.

The EEG is recorded with the patient comatose and jerking. An EMG channel is placed on his right hand. He remains on phenytoin and cardiopressors. Lorazepam and other sedatives are discontinued 5 hours before the recording.

Questions: Is vecuronium required to interpret this study? Is it status epilepticus? What prognostic significance does this pattern have?

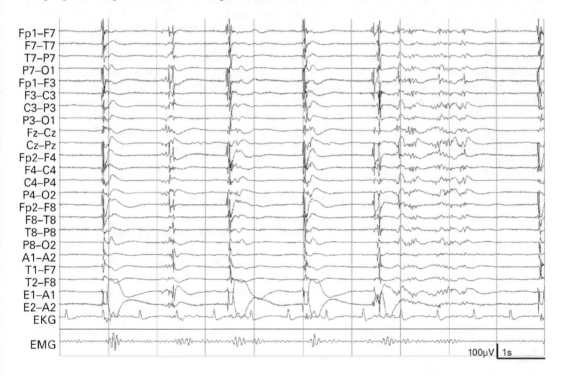

Answers: The recording shows quasi-periodic bursts of multiple spikes occurring on suppressed background activities. The EMG channel shows that multiple spikes precede arm jerks by approximately 200 milliseconds. Because cortical activity precedes EMG changes, vecuronium is not necessary because EMG does not obscure cortical activities. This pattern is consistent with epileptic myoclonus. Its continuous nature is consistent with status myoclonus or myoclonic status epilepticus. It is associated with subsequent death or severe neurologic impairment.

Discussion: *Myoclonic status epilepticus* is defined as continuous myoclonus, in addition to other epileptic seizures that persist for over 30 minutes. The myoclonic seizures can be cortical in origin or arise from subcortical or reticular structures, and both can occur together. Some authors distinguish myoclonic status epilepticus from *status myoclonus*, in which myoclonus, of either epileptic or nonepileptic origin, is not accompanied by other seizure types.

Myoclonic status epilepticus occurs most frequently after cardiac arrest and cerebral anoxia. Depending on the differences in definition and inclusion in various studies, myoclonic status epilepticus occurs after 3–37% of cardiac resuscitations. Out of a combined total of 232 patients studied in the references that follow, myoclonic status epilepticus is observed in 54 (23%). All 54 died subsequent to discovery of myoclonic status epilepticus, despite anticonvulsant therapy.

The poor response to anticonvulsant therapy, both in the ability to stop myoclonus and in the lack of effect in outcome, raises the possibility that, in the spectrum of PEDs versus ictal discharges, myoclonic status epilepticus is an agonal rhythm of diffuse, acute, and severe neuronal injury rather than a seizure state. To withhold anticonvulsant therapy on this interpretation remains controversial. Many physicians continue to treat patients with evidence of cortical myoclonus or mixed seizures, in addition to myoclonus.

In this patient's case, the placement of EMG electrodes on a limb allowed classification of this pattern as an epileptic myoclonus, because cortical discharges preceded and, presumptively, caused myoclonic jerks. If myoclonic jerks occurred simultaneously with cortical discharges, the classification into epileptic (cortical) versus nonepileptic (subcortical) would remain ambiguous, because the short duration, polyphasic spike activity could alternatively be interpreted as muscle artifacts rather than cortical activity. In the latter situation, temporary paralysis could aid in interpretation.

Clinical Pearls

1. Myoclonic status epilepticus is myoclonus and other seizure types persisting beyond 30 minutes.
2. Myoclonic status epilepticus portends severe neuronal injury and death in most subjects if seen after cerebral anoxia.

REFERENCES
1. Krumholz A, Weiss HD: Outcome from coma after cardiopulmonary resuscitation: Relation to seizures myoclonus. Neurology 1988; 38:401–405.
2. Wijdicks EF, Parisi JE, Sharbrough FW: Prognostic value of myoclonus status in comatose survivors of cardiac arrest. Ann Neurol 1994; 35(2):239–243.
3. Young GB, Gilbert JJ, Zochodne DW: The significance of myoclonic status epilepticus in postanoxic coma. Neurology 1990; 40:1843–1848.

INDEX

Page numbers followed by f denote figures.

Other Titles in the Pearls Series®

Duke	**Anesthesia Pearls**	1-56053-495-8
Carabello & Gazes	**Cardiology Pearls, 2nd Edition**	1-56053-403-6
Sahn & Heffner	**Critical Care Pearls, 2nd Edition**	1-56053-224-6
Sahn	**Dermatology Pearls**	1-56053-315-3
Baren & Alpern	**Emergency Medicine Pearls**	1-56053-575-X
Greenberg & Amato	**EMG Pearls**	1-56053-613-6
Jay	**Foot and Ankle Pearls**	1-56053-445-1
Concannon & Hurov	**Hand Pearls**	1-56053-463-X
Danso	**Hematology and Oncology Pearls**	1-56053-577-6
Jones *et al.*	**Hypertension Pearls**	1-56053-583-0
Cunha	**Infectious Disease Pearls**	1-56053-203-3
Heffner & Sahn	**Internal Medicine Pearls, 2nd Edition**	1-56053-404-4
Mercado & Smetana	**Medical Consultation Pearls**	1-56053-504-0
Waclawik & Sutula	**Neurology Pearls**	1-56053-261-0
Gault	**Ophthalmology Pearls**	1-56053-498-2
Heffner & Byock	**Palliative and End-of-Life Pearls**	1-56053-500-8
Inselman	**Pediatric Pulmonary Pearls**	1-56053-350-1
Lennard	**Physical Medicine & Rehabilitation Pearls**	1-56053-455-9
Kolevzon & Stewart	**Psychiatry Pearls**	1-56053-590-3
Silver & Smith	**Rheumatology Pearls**	1-56053-201-7
Berry	**Sleep Medicine Pearls, 2nd Edition**	1-56053-490-7
Eck *et al.*	**Spine Pearls**	1-56053-571-7
Osterhoudt *et al.*	**Toxicology Pearls**	1-56053-614-4
Schluger & Harkin	**Tuberculosis Pearls**	1-56053-156-8
Resnick & Schaeffer	**Urology Pearls**	1-56053-351-X